Hypothermia and Cerebral Ischemia

Hypothermia and Cerebral Ischemia

Mechanisms and Clinical Applications

Edited by

Carolina M. Maier, PhD

*Department of Neurosurgery,
Stanford University School of Medicine, Stanford, CA*

and

Gary K. Steinberg, MD, PhD

*Departments of Neurosurgery and Neurology,
Stanford University School of Medicine, Stanford, CA*

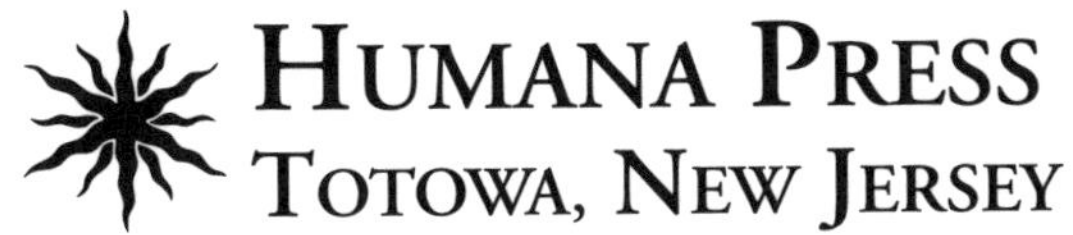

HUMANA PRESS
TOTOWA, NEW JERSEY

Production Editor: Tracy Catanese
Artwork Description: Top Left Panel: Neuronal Immunocytochemistry Composite. Top Right Panel: Magnetic Resonance Image of an Adult Human Brain. Bottom Left Panel: Cerebral Angiogram Highlighting an Aneurysm. Bottom Right Panel: Immunocytochemistry Highlighting Blood Vessels and Inflammatory Cells in an Ischemic Brain. Created by Elizabeth Hoyte and Carolina Maier.

This publication is printed on acid-free paper. ∞
ANSI Z39.48-1984 (American National Standards Institute) Permanence of Paper for Printed Library Materials.

Photocopy Authorization Policy:

Printed in the United States of America. 10 9 8 7 6 5 4 3 2 1
1-59259-653-3 (e-book)

Library of Congress Cataloging-in-Publication Data

Hypothermia and cerebral ischemia : mechanisms and clinical applications / edited by Carolina M. Maier and Gary K. Steinberg.
    p. ; cm.
    Includes bibliographical references and index.
    ISBN 0-89603-660-X
      1. Cerebral ischemia--Treatment. 2. Brain damage--Treatment. 3. Brain--Effect of cold on. 4. Cold--Therapeutic use. I. Maier, Carolina M. II. Steinberg, Gary K.
      [DNLM: 1. Brain Ischemia--therapy. 2. Hypothermia, Induced. 3. Brain Injuries--therapy. 4. Cerebrovascular Accident--therapy. WL 355 H9988 2004]
   RC388.5 H97 2004
   616.8′1--dc21

                                                     2003049949

Preface

Stroke is a global health problem affecting approximately 750,000 people annually in the United States alone and ranks as the third leading cause of death and the most common cause of disability in most developed countries. Traumatic brain injury (TBI) accounts for an estimated 34% of all injury-related deaths in the United States. Stroke and TBI can produce both focal and widespread damage to the brain, which can yield acute and chronic impairments of sensory, motor, and cognitive functions. Because of their enormous medical and socioeconomic impact, a tremendous research investment is being made in the treatment and prevention of stroke and TBI.

Strategies for reducing adverse neurologic outcomes after ischemic or TBI have led to the development of a wide range of neuroprotective agents. However, despite promising results in animal models of stroke and TBI, and extensive testing in randomized clinical trials, no neuroprotective drug has yet proven effective in humans.

In recent years, there has been a resurgence of interest in mild hypothermia as a method of cerebral protection. Although deep hypothermia (below 30°C) is known to be neuroprotective, clinically the benefit is offset by the risks of cardiac arrhythmias and coagulopathies, and by the extensive resources necessary to achieve deep hypothermia, including cardiopulmonary bypass. Alternatively, small decreases in brain temperature (2–5°C below normal brain temperature) are well-tolerated and confer significant neuroprotection in animal models of cerebral ischemia. Indeed, mild hypothermia is one of the most effective neuroprotective therapies in experimental ischemia models, and the feasibility of using mild hypothermia to treat stroke and TBI patients is currently being evaluated in clinical trials. Recently, two prospective, randomized controlled studies demonstrated improved neurologic outcome with mild hypothermic treatment for patients with cardiac arrest from ventricular fibrillation.

Increased understanding of the mechanisms by which mild hypothermia exerts its neuroprotective effects has allowed basic scientists and clinicians to optimize the use of mild hypothermia as a therapeutic strategy. New technological advances are now facilitating the implementation of mild hypothermia in the clinical setting. Knowledge and experience gained from clinical trials around the world have helped develop guidelines for the intraoperative and intensive care management of patients undergoing mild hypothermic treatment.

There is also interest in combining hypothermia with other therapeutic strategies. The rationale for this combination approach is that mild hypothermia could prolong the therapeutic window for neuroprotective agents. Using hypothermia in conjunction with other pharmacological agents for the treatment of acute cerebral ischemia is also discussed in this book, along with future directions in both basic and clinical research.

Hypothermia and Cerebral Ischemia: Mechanisms and Clinical Applications is intended to provide a comprehensive review of mild hypothermia's therapeutic potential, its limitations, and recent developments in both basic and clinical research. We hope that this volume serves to educate clinicians, other health professionals, and basic scientists, as well as promote interest in the study and implementation of mild hypothermia for the treatment of stroke and TBI.

***Carolina M. Maier,** PhD*
***Gary K. Steinberg,** MD, PhD*

Contents

Preface .... *v*

Contributors .... *ix*

1 **Resurgence of Hypothermia as a Treatment for Brain Injury**

  Carolina M. Maier and Gary K. Steinberg *1*

2 **The Effects of Hypothermia and Hyperthermia in Global Cerebral Ischemia**

  Myron D. Ginsberg and Ludmila Belayev *17*

3 **Mild Hypothermia in Experimental Focal Cerebral Ischemia**

  Carolina M. Maier *39*

4 **Hypothermic Protection in Traumatic Brain Injury**

  W. Dalton Dietrich and Miguel A. Pérez-Pinzón *65*

5 **Postischemic Hypothermia Provides Long-Term Neuroprotection in Rodents**

  Frederick Colbourne and Dale Corbett *79*

6 **Combination Therapy With Hypothermia and Pharmaceuticals for the Treatment of Acute Cerebral Ischemia**

  David C. Tong and Midori A. Yenari *93*

7 **Intraoperative and Intensive Care Management of the Patient Undergoing Mild Hypothermia**

  Teresa E. Bell-Stephens, Richard A. Jaffe, and Gary K. Steinberg *103*

8 **Management of Traumatic Brain Injury With Moderate Hypothermia**

  Elad I. Levy and Donald W. Marion *119*

9   Hypothermia: *Clinical Experience in Stroke Patients*
Stefan Schwab and Werner Hacke 145

10   Hypothermia Therapy: *Future Directions
in Research and Clinical Practice*
Wataru Kakuda, Takao Shimizu, and Hiroaki Naritomi 161

Index 179

Contributors

LUDMILA BELAYEV, MD • *Cerebral Vascular Disease Research Center, Department of Neurology, University of Miami School of Medicine, Miami, FL*

TERESA E. BELL-STEPHENS, RN • *Department of Neurosurgery, Stanford Stroke Center, Stanford University School of Medicine, Stanford, CA*

FREDERICK COLBOURNE, PhD • *Department of Psychology, University of Alberta, Edmonton, Canada*

DALE CORBETT, PhD • *Faculty of Medicine, Memorial University of New Foundland, St. John's, Canada*

W. DALTON DIETRICH, PhD • *Miami Project to Cure Paralysis, Neurotrauma Research Center, Departments of Neurological Surgery and Neurology, University of Miami School of Medicine, Miami, FL*

MYRON D. GINSBERG, MD • *Cerebral Vascular Disease Research Center, Department of Neurology, University of Miami School of Medicine, Miami, FL*

WERNER HACKE, MD • *Department of Neurology, University of Heidelberg, Heidelberg, Germany*

RICHARD A. JAFFE, MD, PhD • *Department of Anesthesiology, Stanford University School of Medicine, Stanford, CA*

WATARU KAKUDA, MD • *Stroke Division, Department of Internal Medicine, Hoshigaoka Koseinenkin Hospital, Osaka, Japan*

ELAD I. LEVY, MD • *Department of Neurosurgery and Toshiba Stroke Research Center, School of Medicine and Biomedical Sciences, University of Buffalo, The State University of New York, Buffalo, NY*

CAROLINA M. MAIER, PhD • *Department of Neurosurgery, Stanford Stroke Center, Stanford University School of Medicine, Stanford, CA*

DONALD W. MARION, MD • *Department of Neurosurgery, Boston University School of Medicine, Boston, MA*

HIROAKI NARITOMI, MD • *Cerebrovascular Division, Department of Medicine, National Cardiovascular Center, Osaka, Japan*

MIGUEL A. PÉREZ-PINZÓN, PhD • *Neurotrauma Research Center, Department of Neurology, University of Miami School of Miami School of Medicine, Miami, FL*

STEFAN SCHWAB, MD • *Department of Neurology, University of Heidelberg, Heidelberg, Germany*

TAKAO SHIMIZU, MD • *Department of Medicine, Aino Hospital, Osaka, Japan*

GARY K. STEINBERG, MD, PhD • *Departments of Neurosurgery and Neurology, Stanford Stroke Center, Stanford University School of Medicine, Stanford, CA*

DAVID C. TONG, MD • *Department of Neurology, Stanford Stroke Center, Stanford University School of Medicine, Stanford, CA*

MIDORI A. YENARI, MD • *Departments of Neurosurgery and Neurology, Stanford Stroke Center, Stanford University School of Medicine, Stanford, CA*

1

Resurgence of Hypothermia as a Treatment for Brain Injury

Carolina M. Maier, PhD, *and Gary K. Steinberg,* MD, PhD

INTRODUCTION

Like all homeothermic animals, humans maintain their thermal core temperature within a narrow range despite variations in environmental conditions and endogenous heat production. Thermoregulation is under central nervous system (CNS) control, mainly in the hypothalamus, and body functions are impaired if brain temperature deviates from the normothermic range. With prolonged exposure to an extreme cold challenge in which the thermoregulatory system is overwhelmed, core body temperature falls below the desired temperature range (i.e., hypothermia) and, unless reversed, can lead to death *(1)*. On the other hand, temperature can be modulated in a therapeutic manner to achieve organ protection. Hypothermia-induced protection of tissue has interested scientists and clinicians since the 19th century, when hypothermia was first utilized in the clinical setting as a local anesthetic during surgical procedures.

The use of induced hypothermia as a therapeutic strategy in neurologic emergency care dates back to the early 1940s, when Dr. Temple Fay cooled 124 patients with severe head injury *(2)*. A decade later, Bigelow et al. *(3)* introduced the concept of using hypothermia during cardiac surgical procedures that required circulatory arrest and thus global cerebral ischemia. These studies led to the notion that hypothermia could be used to protect the brain by reducing cerebral metabolism, and nonrandomized trials of induced hypothermia in various neurosurgical subspecialties followed. However, complications such as ventricular fibrillation, acidosis, coagulation disorders, ischemic sensory

From: *Hypothermia and Cerebral Ischemia: Mechanisms and Clinical Applications*
Edited by: C. M. Maier and G. K. Steinberg © Humana Press Inc., Totowa, NJ

neuropathies, increased susceptibility to infections, and even shivering caused hypothermia to fall out of favor. Difficulties in reducing whole body temperature, mainly done by surface cooling and extracorporeal bypass, also limited the applicability of hypothermia. Hence, hypothermia was largely abandoned *(4)*.

In 1987, however, a study by Busto et al. *(5)* showed that small decreases in brain temperature (as little as 2–5°C below normal brain temperature) conferred a marked protective effect against experimental global cerebral ischemia. This finding, as well as subsequent animal studies that modeled neurodegenerative diseases and CNS injury, led to a resurgence of interest in mild hypothermia as a method of cerebral protection.

Mild hypothermia (defined here as reflecting a brain temperature between 33°C and 36°C) is one of the most effective neuroprotective therapies against experimental ischemia that currently exists *(4,6)*. Mild hypothermia has already been used, with varying degrees of success, in the treatment of acute traumatic brain injury *(7,8)*, spinal cord injury *(9,10)*, ischemic stroke *(11,12)*, subarachnoid hemorrhage *(13,14)*, cardiopulmonary arrest *(15)*, hepatic encephalopathy *(16–18)*, perinatal asphyxia *(19,20)*, and infantile viral encephalopathy *(21–23)*. In the past few years there has been renewed interest at the clinical level in developing protocol guidelines for the use of mild hypothermia in patients suffering from acute cerebral ischemia and traumatic brain injury. The efficacy and safety of mild hypothermia are under study in various centers around the world. Preliminary clinical studies have shown that mild hypothermia can be a relatively safe treatment. The feasibility of using mild hypothermia to treat stroke and head injury patients has been evaluated in some clinical trials. With preclinical data suggesting a restricted temporal therapeutic window for the neuroprotective benefit of mild hypothermia, increasing emphasis is being placed on developing techniques and protocols to ensure rapid cooling of patients. Additional multicenter randomized trials are critical to define the indications and limitations for the use of mild hypothermia in the clinical setting.

This chapter gives a general overview on the use of hypothermia as a method of cerebroprotection and highlights some of the issues encountered by both researchers and clinicians regarding the implementation of hypothermia as a therapeutic strategy. The main focus is on two of the leading causes of death and disability in the adult population: stroke and traumatic brain injury. In-depth reports on both basic and clinical aspects of the studies on mild hypothermia are given in the chapters that follow.

EXPERIMENTAL STUDIES

Human neurological disorders can be modeled in animals using standardized procedures that re-create specific pathogenic events and their behavioral outcomes. Animal models are indispensable tools for exploring underlying pathophysiologic mechanisms of neurologic disease and investigation of therapeutic strategies prior to testing them in patients.

The neuroprotective properties of mild hypothermia have been demonstrated in numerous experimental animal models. Research in this area has been conducted for many years, yet the mechanisms of cerebral protection by mild hypothermia remain unclear and continue to be the subject of intense investigation. The neuroprotective effects of mild hypothermia have been attributed to alterations in metabolic rate *(24)*, neurotransmitter release *(25–27)*, activity of protein kinases *(28)*, resynthesis of cellular repair proteins *(29)*, cerebral blood flow *(30)*, preservation of the blood–brain barrier (BBB) *(31)*, attenuation of inflammatory processes *(32,33)*, and decreases in free radical production *(34)*. Although these may all be components of a complex cascade leading to neurologic injury, it has become increasingly clear that the primary mechanism of action of hypothermia may be different at various temperatures as well as under different ischemic and traumatic conditions.

A major difficulty in interpreting study results on mild brain hypothermia stems from the variability in animal models. Global models of cerebral ischemia involve either four-vessel occlusions or forebrain ischemia models (bilateral carotid artery occlusions) and focus mainly on the hippocampus or striatum. Focal models of cerebral ischemia, which typically consist of middle cerebral artery (MCA) blockage, vary in the occlusion method employed (permanent vs transient occlusions), length of occlusion period, the use of normotensive vs hypertensive animal species, and the area of the brain examined. Furthermore, there are variations among these studies as to when hypothermia is instituted: pre-, intra-, or postinsult—as well as for how long a period of time it should be maintained. Mild hypothermia has also been studied in a variety of traumatic brain injury (TBI) models including lateral fluid-percussion brain injury, controlled cortical impact, weight drop, inertial (nonimpact) brain injury, and cold-induced brain trauma *(35)*. All of these models differ in the degree of injury sustained, the affected area, the clinical features modeled, and the outcome measures assessed.

Despite the variability in animal models, the ultimate goals of experimental studies on mild hypothermia are essentially the same:

1. Define the critical period during which mild hypothermia has to be instituted to achieve neuroprotection—the so-called "therapeutic window."
2. Characterize the various physiological changes resulting from mild hypothermia under each experimental ischemic condition including effects on metabolism, cerebral blood flow, and BBB alterations.
3. Elucidate the cellular and molecular mechanisms of hypothermic neuroprotection to optimize the use of mild hypothermia as a neuroprotective strategy.

The importance of using suitable methods of behavioral outcome, and often imaging studies, in addition to histopathology is becoming increasingly recognized as essential in preclinical research *(36,37)*. Determinations of infarct/lesion volumes or neuronal cell counts are not sufficient to detect subtle alterations in pathophysiology that may cause neuronal dysfunction. Such outcome measures are also inadequate to determine the success of a particular neuroprotective strategy, and there is ample evidence regarding the dissociation between behavioral and histological endpoints in animal models of cerebral ischemia *(37)*. Incorporating functional measures as well as longer postischemic survival into experimental protocols increases the validity of animal models and helps reduce the introduction of ineffective therapies into costly clinical trials *(37)*.

The apparent lack of agreement between experimental studies and clinical trials regarding the efficacy of various neuroprotective agents, including mild hypothermia, is further evidence of the importance of choosing appropriate endpoints *(38–40)*. The discrepancies highlight major obstacles in moving from the laboratory bench to the patient bedside. On the experimental side, healthy and relatively young animals are used in a very controlled setting that aims at reducing variables. Both insult and therapy are carefully manipulated. The therapeutic window can be established successfully given strict experimental criteria, and treatment usually can be started and applied without major difficulties— it takes only a few minutes to cool most small animals to the target temperature. In the clinical setting, on the other hand, controlling for the severity of the insult, for associated medical complications, and instituting treatment in a safe and timely fashion is not easily achieved. Time to treatment is an inherent problem in any medical emergency. Using hypothermia as a treatment is complicated further by that fact that with current technology, it takes several hours to cool (and rewarm) a patient safely, which results in adverse side effects or complications not accounted for in the experimental animal setting *(41)*.

The study of mild hypothermia in animal models requires an understanding not only of the clinical features that are to be replicated, but also of species-specific metabolic and behavioral patterns of the animals being used as well as proper endpoints. The successful transition from the laboratory to the clinical arena depends on a continuous exchange of information between clinical investigators and basic scientists.

BRAIN COOLING TECHNIQUES

One of the greatest obstacles in moving from the experimental setting to the study of mild hypothermia in human subjects has been the lack of adequate cooling techniques. Generalized (moderate to deep) hypothermia was initially achieved by surface cooling, which sometimes meant submerging the neurosurgical patient in iced water while he or she was on the operating table *(42)*. This method of cooling was unwieldy, required prolonged anesthesia, did not allow for good temperature control, and led to a variety of medical complications. Several other cooling techniques, including selective brain cooling, were used with various degree of success, but the risk of serious complications and mortality rates were still high by the late 1960s *(4)*. More recently, the feasibility of active core cooling to 32°C (with "core" defined by bladder or rectal temperature) using an extracorporeal heat exchanger was performed in patients with severe head injuries without serious complications, but no beneficial effect of hypothermic therapy on outcome was observed in that small study *(43)*.

At present, systemic surface cooling is the most widely used method to induce and maintain mild hypothermia, but this is now achieved with a water-circulating blanket. While simple and feasible in most patients, this method requires several hours of cooling before the target temperature is reached. To prevent shivering, the patient also has to be sedated, which, combined with prolonged cooling periods, can lead to an increased risk of respiratory infections *(12,44)*. To reduce the cooling period, alternative methods have been developed. Intravenous cooling, for example, can be achieved through infusion of ice-cold saline solution via a central venous catheter or by placing balloons perfused with cold saline in the vessels *(45,46)*. Cooling via transfemoral internal carotid arterial catheterization has also been tested and may be applicable to patients with embolic stroke *(47)*. Recently, the use of several self-contained, transvenous catheter devices has shown promise in safely achieving more rapid cooling of patients *(48–50)*.

How the temperature is measured (i.e., brain vs arterial, venous, tympanic, bladder, or rectal temperature) is also critical, as the core temperature is usually 0.3–1.1°C lower than brain temperature *(51)*. However, it is important to consider that these values may be different in patients with acute cerebral ischemia or trauma.

MILD HYPOTHERMIA AND TRAUMATIC BRAIN INJURY

As mentioned earlier, animal studies have shown that even small decreases in brain temperature reduce the extent of ischemia and TBI-induced neuronal injury, and may improve neuronal survival *(5,52,53)*. Interest in using mild hypothermia as a treatment for clinical severe TBI was renewed in the early 1990s following preliminary studies reporting its efficacy *(54–56)*. In a randomized controlled study *(54)*, 33 severely head-injured patients with persistent intracranial pressure (ICP) >20 mmHg and Glasgow Coma Scale (GCS) scores of 8 or less were treated with mild hypothermia (34°C, 48-h duration). Mild hypothermia reduced ICP, increased cerebral perfusion pressure (CPP), and also significantly reduced the mortality rate compared with results for patients treated under normothermic conditions. Furthermore, mild hypothermia significantly decreased cerebral blood flow, arteriojugular venous oxygen difference, and the cerebral metabolic rate of oxygen ($CMRO_2$). This study suggested that mild hypothermia was a safe and effective method for controlling traumatic intracranial hypertension and could also lower mortality and morbidity rates.

At about the same time, another small randomized study of 40 patients with severe closed head injury (GCS score 3–7) showed that mild hypothermia (brain temperature of 32–33°C, 24-h duration) significantly reduced ICP (40%) and CBF (26%) during the cooling period *(56)*. Compared to the normothermia group, the mean $CMRO_2$ in the hypothermia group was lower during cooling but higher 5 d after injury. By 3 mo postinsult, there was a trend toward better outcome in patients treated with hypothermia. Similar findings came from a third preliminary study in which 46 patients with severe TBI were treated with either mild hypothermia (32–33°C, 48-h duration) or normothermia *(55)*. Hypothermia-treated patients showed improved neurologic outcome with minimal toxicity, and the authors concluded that phase III testing of hypothermia in patients with severe head injury was warranted.

Several studies on mild hypothermia and TBI employing human subjects followed, with mixed results. In a prospective randomized, single-center, controlled trial, Marion et al. *(8)* compared the effects of hypothermia (32–33°C, 24-h duration) and normothermia in 82 patients with severe closed head injuries (GCS scores of 3–7). They showed that, at 3–6 mo, mild hypothermia significantly improved the outcome of patients with admission GCS scores of 5–7 (but not lower). However, there was no statistically significant improvement of hypothermia-treated patients at 12 mo postinsult compared with the normothermia-treated group, suggesting that hypothermia may have simply accelerated neurologic recovery. These results were confirmed by Shiozaki et al. *(57,58)*, who showed that mild hypothermia was ineffective in patients with severe TBI. In that study, 45 patients in the hypothermia-treated group were exposed to mild hypothermia (34°C, 48-h duration) followed by rewarming at 1°C per day for 3 d, whereas patients in the normothermic group ($n = 46$) were kept at 37°C for 5 d. The authors found no difference in clinical outcome at 3 mo postinjury between the two temperature groups and concluded that mild hypothermia should not be used for the treatment of severely head-injured patients in whom ICP could be maintained at <25 mmHg by conventional therapies.

Another large prospective, randomized multicenter trial was recently published and echoed results from the studies just mentioned *(7)*. In this trial, a total of 392 patients with severe TBI (GCS scores of 3–8) were randomly assigned for treatment with hypothermia (core temperature of 33°C, 48-h duration), which was initiated within 6 h after injury by means of surface cooling, or with normothermia. The results showed poor outcome in both temperature groups and no difference in mortality rate. There was, however, a beneficial effect in patients younger than 45 yr of age in whom hypothermia was present on admission. While hypothermia was able to reduce the ICP in patients with intracranial hypertension, hypothermia-treated patients had a higher rate of complications and longer hospital stays than those in the normothermic group. Two recently published meta-analyses failed to demonstrate a benefit of mild hypothermic treatment for patients with traumatic brain injury *(59,60)*.

Discrepancies between results from the preliminary studies and the larger, multicenter trials remain to be elucidated. Significant intercenter variance in patient management (fluids, mean arterial blood pressure, ICP, and CPP) and treatment may have adversely affected the results of one of these trials (The National Acute Brain Injury Study: Hypothermia) *(61)*. Despite the overall negative findings, however, it is quite possible that certain subgroups of patients may benefit from treatment with mild hypothermia.

MILD HYPOTHERMIA
AND TREATMENT OF ACUTE ISCHEMIC STROKE

Extensive studies in both global and focal models of cerebral ischemia have established the neuroprotective effects of mild hypothermia in the experimental setting *(4)*. In the mid-1990s, those studies led to the investigation of the therapeutic value of mild hypothermia in stroke patients. In a prospective study of 390 stroke patients who were admitted to the hospital within 6 h after stroke, Reith et al. examined the relationship between body temperature on admission with acute stroke and various indices of stroke severity and outcome *(62)*. Their results showed reduced mortality, smaller infarcts, and better outcome in patients with mild hypothermia on admission. More importantly, they showed that these outcome parameters were worse in patients with *hyper*thermia. Similar results were obtained from a study by Azzimondi et al. *(63)*, who showed that fever in the first week after stroke was an independent predictor of poor outcome. This was not surprising to the basic scientists, as laboratory investigations had shown the adverse effects of fever of even moderate degree in terms not only of functional outcomes, but also histologic and neurochemical injury *(4,64–66)*. However, in these clinical studies correlating body temperature after stroke and outcome, it might be argued that increased severity of stroke caused elevated temperature rather than being the consequence of it.

It is now well recognized that hyperthermia should be avoided in ischemic stroke patients *(67–69)* and possibly in a variety of acute neurosurgical diseases. Unfortunately, fever is still a very common event following stroke and TBI, as well as subarachnoid hemorrhage (SAH) *(70)*. Hyperthermia should be treated as soon as possible following an acute ischemic stroke, but the aggressive lowering of temperature below the normal physiologic range is more controversial.

In an attempt to determine whether there was a causal relationship between hypothermia and better neurological outcome following stroke, Schwab et al. *(44)* studied a group of 25 patients who had suffered severe ischemic stroke in the MCA territory. Mild hypothermia (33°C, 48- to 72-h duration) was induced using cooling blankets. Results from that study showed that mild hypothermia was helpful in controlling critically elevated ICP values, reduced morbidity, and improved long-term clinical outcome compared with historical controls. Although no severe side effects of hypothermia were detected, 40% of hypothermic patients developed pneumonia.

The same group evaluated the safety and feasibility of mild hypothermia for the treatment of acute ischemic stroke in a follow-up study *(12)*. Fifty prospective patients with cerebral infarction involving the complete MCA territory were treated with mild hypothermia (33°C, 24- to 72-h duration). Although the use of mild hypothermia was found to be feasible in patients with acute stroke, the treatment was associated with several adverse effects, including thrombocytopenia, bradycardia, and pneumonia. This study also showed that most deaths occurred during rewarming as a result of excessive ICP increases, leading the authors to conclude that longer duration of rewarming might help reduce mortality. Of note in the above studies is the induction time of mild hypothermia. In the first study *(44)*, hypothermia was induced 14 ± 7 h after stroke onset, compared to an induction time of 22 ± 9 h in the follow-up report *(12)*. This is important because, in animal studies, the therapeutic window for mild hypothermia is believed to be within 60–90 min after induction of focal cerebral ischemia, although more delayed induction has also been shown to be beneficial with prolonged hypothermic treatment *(4,71,72)*. In human studies, it was speculated that hypothermia treatment would be most beneficial if applied within 0–6 h from stroke symptom onset *(44)*.

Recently, two landmark prospective randomized controlled studies were published demonstrating the benefit of mild hypothermia in improving neurologic outcome in patients suffering cardiac arrest from ventricular fibrillation *(73,74)*.

In the European study *(74)*, patients who had been resuscitated after cardiac arrest from ventricular fibrillation were randomized to either therapeutic hypothermia over 24 h or normothermia. The median interval between restoration of spontaneous circulation and attainment of the target temperature 32°–34°C was 8 h. Favorable neurologic outcome at 6 mo, defined as good recovery or moderate disability, was found in 75 of 136 (55%) of patients in the hypothermia group compared with 54 of 137 (39%) of patients in the normothermia group ($p = 0.009$). Mortality at 6 mo was also reduced in the hypothermia group (41% vs 55% for normothermia) ($p = 0.02$). There was no difference in the complication rate between groups.

The Australian study *(73)* randomly assigned 77 patients with ventricular fibrillation cardiac arrest to hypothermia (33°C) or normothermia. Patients were cooled within 2 h after return to spontaneous circulation and maintained at that temperature for 12 h. Forty-nine percent (21/43) of the hypothermia-treated patients had a good outcome, defined as discharged home or to a rehabilitation facility compared with 26% (9/34) of the normothermia group ($p = 0.046$). There was no difference in the frequency of adverse effects between groups.

The need to cool patients quickly while at the same time reducing complication rates has led to the development of simpler methods of rapidly inducing and maintaining hypothermia. More modest hypothermia can now be achieved in awake patients with acute stroke by surface cooling with the "forced air" method in combination with pethidine to treat shivering *(75)*, and several intravenous vascular cooling techniques look encouraging *(48–50)*.

Another promising therapeutic approach in both basic and clinical research is to combine mild hypothermia with various pharmacological agents. One recently published study examined the feasibility and safety of adjunct mild hypothermia in patients with acute ischemic stroke undergoing thrombolysis *(76)*. The mean time from symptom onset to tissue plasminogen activator (t-PA) infusion was 3.1 ± 1.4 h and from symptom onset to initiation of hypothermia it was 6.2 ± 1.3 h. The target temperature was achieved within 2–6.5 h, while rewarming required an average of 22.6 ± 15.6 h. Ten patients were kept hypothermic (32°C) for 12–72 h while another nine were kept normothermic. Hypothermia was well tolerated by most patients and there were no significant differences in minor or major complication rates between the two temperature groups. Although there was a tendency toward better outcomes in the hypothermic group, no conclusions could be drawn regarding the efficacy of hypothermia.

Combination therapy remains a viable and encouraging alternative. However, this requires careful identification of patient subgroups and detailed understanding of the special pathology involved so that individual treatment can be tailored accordingly. The therapeutic window for mild hypothermia remains to be defined in patient subgroups. Standardized guidelines for treatment and patient care, including the cooling method used, also need to be addressed. This can be accomplished only with carefully monitored multicenter, randomized, controlled trials. Fundamental, preclinical research is also critical to enhance our understanding of the pathophysiology involved and, hence, optimize treatment strategies. Both clinicians and basic scientists remain optimistic that over the next decade mild hypothermia will emerge as a major effective therapeutic advance for patients with acute neurologic injury.

REFERENCES

1. Crawshaw L., Grahn D., Wollmuth L., and Simpson L. (1985) Central nervous regulation of body temperature in vertebrates: comparative aspects. *Pharmacol. Ther.* **30,** 19–30.
2. Fay T. (1943) Observations on generalized refrigeration in cases of severe cerebral trauma. *Assoc. Res. Nerv. Ment. Dis. Proc.* **24,** 611–619.
3. Bigelow W. D., Lindsay W. K., and Greenwood W. F. (1950) Hypothermia. Its possible role in cardiac surgery: an investigation of factors governing survival in dogs at low body temperatures. *Ann. Surg.* **132,** 849–866.
4. Ginsberg M. D., Sternau L. L., Globus M. Y., Dietrich W. D., and Busto R. (1992) Therapeutic modulation of brain temperature: relevance to ischemic brain injury. *Cerebrovasc. Brain Metab. Rev.* **4,** 189–225.
5. Busto R., Dietrich W. D., Globus M. Y., Valdes I., Scheinberg P., and Ginsberg M. D. (1987) Small differences in intraischemic brain temperature critically determine the extent of ischemic neuronal injury. *J. Cereb. Blood Flow Metab.* **7,** 729–738.
6. Barone F. C., Feuerstein G. Z., and White R. F. (1997) Brain cooling during transient focal ischemia provides complete neuroprotection. *Neurosci. Biobehav. Rev.* **21,** 31–44.
7. Clifton G. L., Miller E. R., Choi S. C., et al. (2001) Lack of effect of induction of hypothermia after acute brain injury. *N. Engl. J. Med.* **344,** 556–563.
8. Marion D. W., Penrod L. E., Kelsey S. F., et al. (1997) Treatment of traumatic brain injury with moderate hypothermia. *N. Engl. J. Med.* **336,** 540–546.
9. Negrin J., Jr. (1973) Spinal cord hypothermia in the neurosurgical management of the acute and chronic post-traumatic paraplegic patient. *Paraplegia* **10,** 336–343.
10. Tator C. H. and Deecke L. (1973) Therapeutic value of local perfusion for acute spinal cord trauma. *Trans. Am. Neurol. Assoc.* **98,** 107–109.
11. Schwab S., Schwarz S., Aschoff A., Keller E., and Hacke W. (1998) Moderate hypothermia and brain temperature in patients with severe middle cerebral artery infarction. *Acta Neurochir. Suppl.* **71,** 131–134.

12. Schwab S., Georgiadis D., Berrouschot J., Schellinger P. D., Graffagnino C., and Mayer S. A. (2001) Feasibility and safety of moderate hypothermia after massive hemispheric infarction. *Stroke* **32,** 2033–2035.

13. Komatsu Y., Fujita K., and Iguchi M. (2000) Mild hypothermia as a protective therapy for severe subarachnoid hemorrhage. *Surg. Cereb. Stroke* **29,** 16–20.

14. Nagao S., Irie K., Kawai N., et al. (2000) Protective effect of mild hypothermia on symptomatic vasospasm: a preliminary report. *Acta Neurochir. Suppl.* **76,** 547–550.

15. Bernard S. A., Jones B. M., and Horne M. K. (1997) Clinical trial of induced hypothermia in comatose survivors of out-of-hospital cardiac arrest. *Ann. Emerg. Med.* **30,** 146–153.

16. Jalan R., Damink S. W., Deutz N. E., Lee A., and Hayes P. C. (1999) Moderate hypothermia for uncontrolled intracranial hypertension in acute liver failure. *Lancet* **354,** 1164–1168.

17. Jalan R., Olde Damink S. W., Deutz N. E., Hayes P. C., and Lee A. (2001) Restoration of cerebral blood flow autoregulation and reactivity to carbon dioxide in acute liver failure by moderate hypothermia. *Hepatology* **34,** 50–54.

18. Blei A. (2000) Hypothermia for fulminant hepatic failure: a cool approach to a burning problem. *Liver Transplant.* **6,** 245–247.

19. Azzopardi D., Robertson N. J., Cowan F. M., Rutherford M. A., Rampling M., and Edwards A. D. (2000) Pilot study of treatment with whole body hypothermia for neonatal encephalopathy. *Pediatrics* **106,** 684–694.

20. Gunn A. J. (2000) Cerebral hypothermia for prevention of brain injury following perinatal asphyxia. *Curr. Opin. Pediatr.* **12,** 111–115.

21. Nakashita Y. and Aoki M. (2000) [Mild brain hypothermia for influenza encephalitis/encephalopathy and its significance]. Nippon Rinsho **58,** 2333–2337.

22. Munakata M., Kato R., Yokoyama H., et al. (2000) Combined therapy with hypothermia and anticytokine agents in influenza A encephalopathy. *Brain Dev.* **22,** 373–377.

23. Ohtsuki N., Kimura S., Nezu A., and Aihara Y. (2000) [Effects of mild hypothermia and steroid pulse combination therapy on acute encephalopathy associated with influenza virus infection: report of two cases]. *No To Hattatsu* **32,** 318–322.

24. Chopp M., Knight R., Tidwell C. D., Helpern J. A., Brown E., and Welch K. M. (1989) The metabolic effects of mild hypothermia on global cerebral ischemia and recirculation in the cat: comparison to normothermia and hyperthermia. *J. Cereb. Blood Flow Metab.* **9,** 141–148.

25. Busto R., Globus M. Y., Dietrich W. D., Martinez E., Valdes I., and Ginsberg M. D. (1989) Effect of mild hypothermia on ischemia-induced release of neurotransmitters and free fatty acids in rat brain. *Stroke* **20,** 904–910.

26. Globus M. Y., Busto R., Dietrich W. D., Martinez E., Valdes I., and Ginsberg M. D. (1988) Intra-ischemic extracellular release of dopamine and glutamate is associated with striatal vulnerability to ischemia. *Neurosci. Lett.* **91,** 36–40.

27. Lo E. H., Steinberg G. K., Panahian N., Maidment N. T., and Newcomb R. (1993) Profiles of extracellular amino acid changes in focal cerebral ischaemia: effects of mild hypothermia. *Neurol. Res.* **15,** 281–287.

28. Cardell M., Boris-Moller F., and Wieloch T. (1991) Hypothermia prevents the ischemia-induced translocation and inhibition of protein kinase C in the rat striatum. *J. Neurochem.* **57,** 1814–1817.

29. Yamashita K., Eguchi Y., Kajiwara K., and Ito H. (1991) Mild hypothermia ameliorates ubiquitin synthesis and prevents delayed neuronal death in the gerbil hippocampus. *Stroke* **22,** 1574–1581.

30. Lo E. H. and Steinberg G. K. (1992) Effects of hypothermia on evoked potentials, magnetic resonance imaging, and blood flow in focal ischemia in rabbits. *Stroke* **23,** 889–893.

31. Dietrich W. D., Busto R., Halley M., and Valdes I. (1990) The importance of brain temperature in alterations of the blood-brain barrier following cerebral ischemia. *J. Neuropathol. Exp. Neurol.* **49,** 486–497.

32. Han H. S., Qiao Y., Karabiyikoglu M., Giffard R. G., and Yenari M. A. (2002) Influence of mild hypothermia on inducible nitric oxide synthase expression and reactive nitrogen production in experimental stroke and inflammation. *J. Neurosci.* **22,** 3921–3928.

33. Wang G. J., Deng H. Y., Maier C. M., Sun G. H., and Yenari M. A. (2002) Mild hypothermia decreases ICAM-1 expression, neutrophil infiltration and microglia/monocyte accumulation following experimental stroke. *Neuroscience* **114,** 1081–1090.

34. Maier C. M., Sun G. H., Cheng D., Yenari M. A., Chan P. H., and Steinberg G. K. (2002) Effects of mild hypothermia on superoxide anion production, superoxide dismutase expression, and activity following transient focal cerebral ischemia. *Neurobiol. Dis.* **11,** 28–42.

35. Dietrich W. D. (1996) Nonpharmacological strategies: moderate hypothermia. In *Neurotrauma* (Narayan R. K., Wilberger J. E., and Povlishock J. T., eds.), McGraw-Hill, New York, pp. 1491–1506.

36. Schallert T., Leasure J. L., and Kolb B. (2000) Experience-associated structural events, subependymal cellular proliferative activity, and functional recovery after injury to the central nervous system. *J. Cereb. Blood Flow Metab.* **20,** 1513–1528.

37. Corbett D. and Nurse S. (1998) The problem of assessing effective neuroprotection in experimental cerebral ischemia. *Prog. Neurobiol.* **54,** 531–548.

38. Dirnagl U., Iadecola C., and Moskowitz M. A. (1999) Pathobiology of ischaemic stroke: an integrated view. *Trends Neurosci.* **22,** 391–397.

39. Alonso de Lecinana M., Diez-Tejedor E., Carceller F., and Roda J. M. (2001) Cerebral ischemia: from animal studies to clinical practice. Should the methods be reviewed? *Cerebrovasc. Dis.* **11(Suppl. 1),** 20–30.

40. DeVries A. C., Nelson R. J., Traystman R. J., and Hurn P. D. (2001) Cognitive and behavioral assessment in experimental stroke research: will it prove useful? *Neurosci. Biobehav. Rev.* **25,** 325–342.

41. Grotta J. (2002) Neuroprotection is unlikely to be effective in humans using current trial designs. *Stroke* **33,** 306–307.

42. Gardner W. J., Wasmuth C. E., and Hale D. E. (1956) A method for converting an operating table into a refrigeration trough. *J. Neurosurg.* **13,** 122–123.

43. Piepgras A., Roth H., Schurer L., et al. (1998) Rapid active internal core cooling for induction of moderate hypothermia in head injury by use of an extracorporeal heat exchanger. *Neurosurgery* **42,** 311–317; discussion 317–318.

44. Schwab S., Schwarz S., Spranger M., Keller E., Bertram M., and Hacke W. (1998) Moderate hypothermia in the treatment of patients with severe middle cerebral artery infarction. *Stroke* **29,** 2461–2466.

45. Rajek A., Greif R., Sessler D. I., Baumgardner J., Laciny S., and Bastanmehr H. (2000) Core cooling by central venous infusion of ice-cold (4 degrees C and 20 degrees C) fluid: isolation of core and peripheral thermal compartments. *Anesthesiology* **93,** 629–637.

46. Georgiadis D., Schwarz S., Kollmar R., and Schwab S. (2001) Endovascular cooling for moderate hypothermia in patients with acute stroke: first results of a novel approach. *Stroke* **32,** 2550–2553.
47. Schwartz A. E., Stone J. G., Pile-Spellman J., et al. (1996) Selective cerebral hypothermia by means of transfemoral internal carotid artery catheterization. *Radiology* **201,** 571–572.
48. Steinberg G. K., Bell-Stephens T., Shuer L. M., et al. (2003) Comparison of endovascular cooling to surface-cooling during unruptured cerebral aneurysm repair. *Stroke* **34,** 246.
49. Steinberg G. K., Ogilvy C. S., Giannotta S., et al. (2001) Multi-center trial of a venous catheter for temperature control during aneurysm surgery: preliminary review of the T. C. A. S study. *Annu. Meet. Congr. Neurol. Surg. Prog.* **51,** 255.
50. De Georgia M. A., Abou-Chebl A., Krieger D. W., Andrefsky J. C., Sila C. A., and Furlan A. J. (2002) Endovascular cooling for patients with acute ischemic stroke. *Stroke* **33,** 271.
51. Henker R. A., Brown S. D., and Marion D. W. (1998) Comparison of brain temperature with bladder and rectal temperatures in adults with severe head injury. *Neurosurgery* **42,** 1071–1075.
52. Globus M. Y., Alonso O., Dietrich W. D., Busto R., and Ginsberg M. D. (1995) Glutamate release and free radical production following brain injury: effects of posttraumatic hypothermia. *J. Neurochem.* **65,** 1704–1711.
53. Huh P. W., Belayev L., Zhao W., Koch S., Busto R., and Ginsberg M. D. (2000) Comparative neuroprotective efficacy of prolonged moderate intraischemic and postischemic hypothermia in focal cerebral ischemia. *J. Neurosurg.* **92,** 91–99.
54. Shiozaki T., Sugimoto H., Taneda M., et al. (1993) Effect of mild hypothermia on uncontrollable intracranial hypertension after severe head injury. *J. Neurosurg.* **79,** 363–368.
55. Clifton G. L., Allen S., Barrodale P., et al. (1993) A phase II study of moderate hypothermia in severe brain injury. *J. Neurotrauma* **10,** 263–271; discussion 273.
56. Marion D. W., Obrist W. D., Carlier P. M., Penrod L. E., and Darby J. M. (1993) The use of moderate therapeutic hypothermia for patients with severe head injuries: a preliminary report. *J. Neurosurg.* **79,** 354–362.
57. Shiozaki T., Kato A., Taneda M., et al. (1999) Little benefit from mild hypothermia therapy for severely head injured patients with low intracranial pressure. *J. Neurosurg.* **91,** 185–191.
58. Shiozaki T., Hayakata T., Taneda M., et al. (2001) A multicenter prospective randomized controlled trial of the efficacy of mild hypothermia for severely head injured patients with low intracranial pressure. Mild Hypothermia Study Group in Japan. *J. Neurosurg.* **94,** 50–54.
59. Harris O. A., Colford J. M., Jr., Good M. C., and Matz P. G. (2002) The role of hypothermia in the management of severe brain injury: a meta-analysis. *Arch. Neurol.* **59,** 1077–1083.
60. Gadkary C. S., Alderson P., and Signorini D. F. (2002) Therapeutic hypothermia for head injury. *Cochrane Database Syst. Rev.* CD001048.
61. Clifton G. L., Choi S. C., Miller E. R., et al. (2001) Intercenter variance in clinical trials of head trauma—experience of the National Acute Brain Injury Study: Hypothermia. *J. Neurosurg.* **95,** 751–755.
62. Reith J., Jorgensen H. S., Pedersen P. M., et al. (1996) Body temperature in acute stroke: relation to stroke severity, infarct size, mortality, and outcome. *Lancet* **347,** 422–425.

63. Azzimondi G., Bassein L., Nonino F., et al. (1995) Fever in acute stroke worsens prognosis. *Stroke* **26,** 2040–2043.
64. Kim Y., Busto R., Dietrich W. D., Kraydieh S., and Ginsberg M. D. (1996) Delayed postischemic hyperthermia in awake rats worsens the histopathological outcome of transient focal cerebral ischemia. *Stroke* **27,** 2274–2280; discussion 2281.
65. Memezawa H., Zhao Q., Smith M. L., and Siesjo B. K. (1995) Hyperthermia nullifies the ameliorating effect of dizocilpine maleate (MK-801) in focal cerebral ischemia. *Brain Res.* **670,** 48–52.
66. Dietrich W. D., Busto R., Valdes I., and Loor Y. (1990) Effects of normothermic versus mild hyperthermic forebrain ischemia in rats. *Stroke* **21,** 1318–1325.
67. Ginsberg M. D. and Busto R. (1998) Combating hyperthermia in acute stroke: a significant clinical concern. *Stroke* **29,** 529–534.
68. Kammersgaard L. P., Jorgensen H. S., Rungby J. A., et al. (2002) Admission body temperature predicts long-term mortality after acute stroke: the Copenhagen Stroke Study. *Stroke* **33,** 1759–1762.
69. Kilpatrick M. M., Lowry D. W., Firlik A. D., Yonas H., and Marion D. W. (2000) Hyperthermia in the neurosurgical intensive care unit. *Neurosurgery* **47,** 850–855; discussion 855–856.
70. Marion D. W. (2001) Therapeutic moderate hypothermia and fever. *Curr. Pharm. Des.* **7,** 1533–1536.
71. Maier C. M., Ahern K., Cheng M. L., Lee J. E., Yenari M. A., and Steinberg G. K. (1998) Optimal depth and duration of mild hypothermia in a focal model of transient cerebral ischemia: effects on neurologic outcome, infarct size, apoptosis, and inflammation. *Stroke* **29,** 2171–2180.
72. Corbett D., Nurse S., and Colbourne F. (1997) Hypothermic neuroprotection. A global ischemia study using 18- to 20-month-old gerbils. *Stroke* **28,** 2238–2242.
73. Bernard S. A., Gray T. W., Buist M. D., et al. (2002) Treatment of comatose survivors of out-of-hospital cardiac arrest with induced hypothermia. *N. Engl. J. Med.* **346,** 557–563.
74. (No authors listed) (2002) Mild therapeutic hypothermia to improve the neurologic outcome after cardiac arrest. *N. Engl. J. Med.* **346,** 549–556.
75. Kammersgaard L. P., Rasmussen B. H., Jorgensen H. S., Reith J., Weber U., and Olsen T. S. (2000) Feasibility and safety of inducing modest hypothermia in awake patients with acute stroke through surface cooling: a case-control study: the Copenhagen Stroke Study. *Stroke* **31,** 2251–2256.
76. Krieger D. W., De Georgia M. A., Abou-Chebl A., et al. (2001) Cooling for acute ischemic brain damage (cool aid): an open pilot study of induced hypothermia in acute ischemic stroke. *Stroke* **32,** 1847–1854.

2

The Effects of Hypothermia and Hyperthermia in Global Cerebral Ischemia

Myron D. Ginsberg, MD,
and Ludmila Belayev, MD

INTRODUCTION

The colorful early history of therapeutic hypothermia has been reviewed elsewhere *(1)*. Its first documented application was as a local anesthetic during surgical procedures. Early in the 20th century, head injury, tumors, and other conditions were treated using local and generalized cooling *(2,3)*. Clinical descriptions note retrograde amnesia at temperatures below 34°C, dysarthria at 34°C, aphasia at 27°C, loss of the pupillary light reflex at 26°C, and the common occurrence of sudden cardiac failure, perhaps attributable to ventricular fibrillation *(4)*. During World War II, the Nazis exposed concentration camp victims to inhumane hypothermia experimentation; these brutal atrocities have been reviewed recently *(5)*.

In cardiac surgical procedures requiring the interruption of circulation, hypothermia was introduced to confer protection against cerebral ischemia and was eventually applied via pump oxygenation and extra-corporeal cooling *(6)*. Hypothermia was also used to mitigate cerebral ischemia resulting from vascular occlusion or hypotension in the course of cerebral aneurysm clipping or the resection of arteriovenous malformations *(7)*. Temperatures as low as 4–15°C were used in cardiac bypass procedures *(8)*. Profound systemic hypothermia, however, was typically associated with severe medical complications including ventricular fibrillation and other cardiac arrhythmias, hypotension, acidosis, coagulopathies, and suppression of immunological function *(9,10)*.

From: *Hypothermia and Cerebral Ischemia: Mechanisms and Clinical Applications*
Edited by: C. M. Maier and G. K. Steinberg © Humana Press Inc., Totowa, NJ

Nonetheless, the enthusiasm for profound hypothermia was bolstered by experimental studies revealing progressive linear declines in cerebral oxygen utilization with decreasing temperature *(11,12)*, and by demonstrations that profound hypothermia was neuroprotective in canine models of ischemia and cerebral contusion *(13,14)*. Selective brain-cooling methods such as cold carotid artery perfusion were considered as a means of avoiding systemic complications, but mortality remained high *(15)*. This might have been attributable in part to alterations of vascular tone provoked by the perfusate *(16)*. Nonetheless, remarkable experimental results emerged from selective brain cooling to 14–15°C: monkeys with 45 min of complete cerebral circulatory arrest recovered without deficits when so cooled *(17)*.

MODULATION OF ISCHEMIC INJURY BY MILD TO MODERATE HYPOTHERMIA

In studies conducted in the 1960s in a model of complete brain ischemia in rabbits, it was shown that the duration of tolerable ischemia compatible with complete functional and histological recovery increased continuously with declining temperature, and could be extended fivefold by reducing temperature from 37°C to 25°C *(18)*. Other workers showed that a decrease of body temperature of only 1–3°C reduced the degree of brain energy metabolite depletion and acidosis in a model of carotid ligation and hypoxia *(19)*.

These observations emphasize the necessity for stringent control of body temperature in the conduct of animal ischemia experiments. The more specific need to monitor and regulate brain temperature, however, was not initially appreciated. Experimental hypoxia–ischemia studies conducted prior to the mid-1980s typically controlled the rectal temperature of their animal preparations but failed to monitor or regulate brain temperature. This situation changed when our group serendipitously observed that rats with global ischemia had less severe neuropathology when their scalp tissues had been reflected for electroencephalographic (EEG) monitoring than did animals with intact scalps—suggesting that the former setting might have led to cranial cooling (study described in Vibulsresth et al. *[20]*). Indeed, by separately monitoring rectal, temporalis muscle, and brain (striatal) temperature, we documented spontaneous, variable declines in cranial and brain temperature during a 20-min global ischemic insult *(21)*. These observations, we hypothesized, accounted for much of the variability noted in previously published animal studies of global ischemia (e.g., Smith et al. *[22]*) and emphasized the need for independent control of both rectal and cranial temperatures.

To study this problem carefully, we conducted experiments in which anesthetized Wistar rats received a 20-min global forebrain ischemic insult by a modification of the four-vessel occlusion method *(23)*. Brain temperature was monitored by a thermocouple inserted stereotaxically into the striatum, and striatal temperature was regulated by a high-intensity lamp positioned over the head *(21)*. In all animals, rectal temperature was separately regulated at 37°C. Brain temperature, however, was intentionally thermostated during the ischemic insult at 33, 34, 36, or 39°C. Following 3-d survival, histopathology in the normothermic group (36°C intraischemic brain temperature) revealed prominent ischemic neuronal pathology in the dorsolateral and central striatum, as well as a marked loss of CA1 pyramidal neurons of the hippocampus (**Fig. 1**). In animals with intraischemic brain cooling to 33–34°C, the extent of these neuronal changes was markedly reduced in both hippocampus and striatum; animals with intraischemic brain temperatures of 30°C had even more pronounced neuroprotection *(21)*. This study thus established that effective hypothermic neuroprotection was possible by intraischemic brain temperature reductions as small as 2°C, and it emphasized that brain temperature is a crucial determinant of ischemic injury and must be separately monitored and regulated to obtain interpretable data from animal experiments. As temporalis muscle temperature correlated highly with brain temperature *(24)*, it could be monitored in lieu of a direct brain thermocouple insertion provided that calibration curves were specifically established under the conditions of each experiment *(25)*.

Other laboratories have repeatedly confirmed the determinative influence of small decrements of brain temperature on the histological outcome of global ischemia. Thus, a 2°C body temperature reduction in ischemic gerbils led to complete protection of CA1 hippocampal neurons *(26)*. In the rat model of bilateral carotid artery occlusions and hypotension, temperature reductions to 35°C protected against selective neuronal necrosis in vulnerable regions *(27,28)*. Selective brain cooling during and following a prolonged (30-min) period of global ischemia in rats reduced cortical damage *(29)*. In studies of ischemic insults in which the temperature was not controlled and a spontaneous decline of brain temperature was permitted, protection of hippocampal

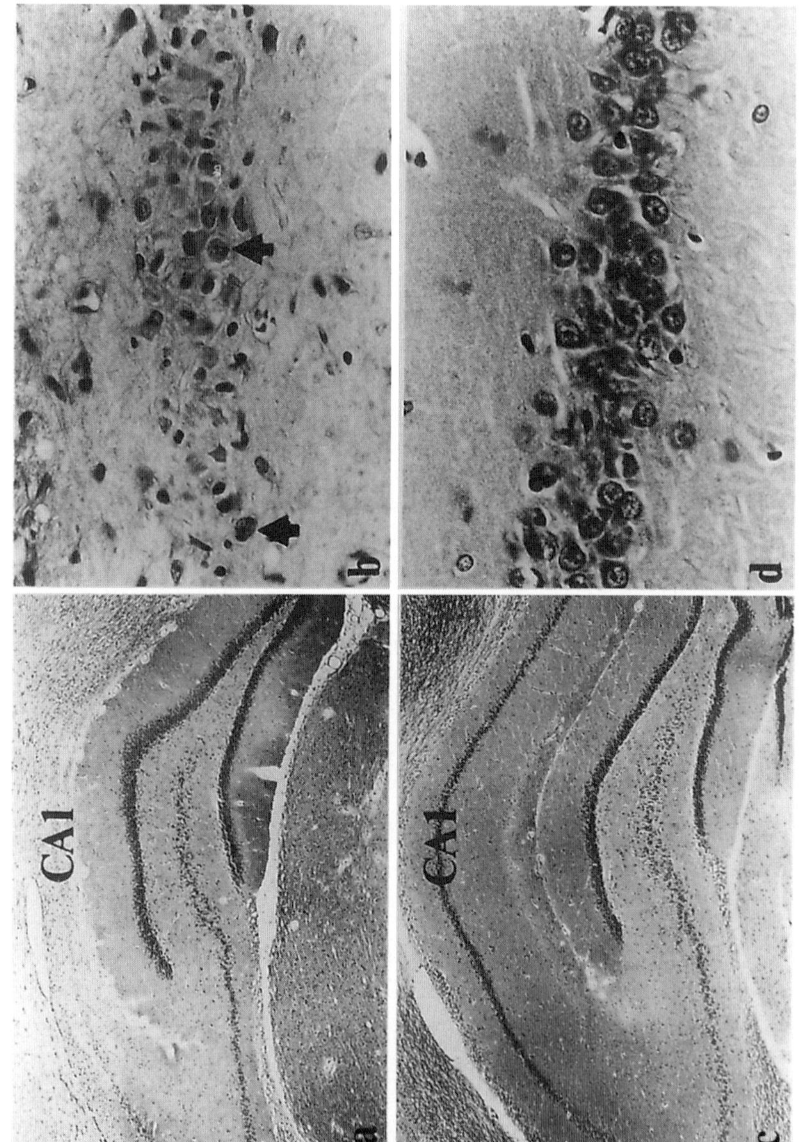

Fig. 1.

neurons was demonstrated relative to the situation in which the brain was held at preischemic, normothermic levels *(27,30,31)*. Moderate hypothermia (32–33°C) was also able to increase survival, abolish seizures, and diminish the extent of pathological alterations in the setting of global ischemia compounded by hyperglycemia *(32)*.

Moderate hypothermia has also proven neuroprotective in animal models of cardiac arrest and cardiopulmonary bypass. In a canine cardiac arrest model, hypothermia to 34°C produced by ice water immersion of the head during the period of arrest and 1 h thereafter led to histopathological improvement *(33)*. These results were confirmed by a later study in which dogs were cooled for 1 h postarrest to 30–34°C; in that study, however, deeper hypothermia (15°C) worsened outcome *(9)*. If cooling was delayed by 15 min after reperfusion, the beneficial effect of resuscitative hypothermia after cardiac arrest in dogs was lost *(34)*. In another canine study, a temperature change of even 1–2°C within the 37–39°C range significantly altered neurological outcome and histopathology in a model of complete cerebral ischemia produced by arterial hypotension plus intracranial hypertension *(35)*. Selective brain cooling to 25–30°C reduced neuronal injury in a cat model of cardiac arrest and resuscitation *(36)*. In a pig cardiopulmonary bypass study, neuronal degeneration and astrocytic swelling were prevented by moderate hypothermia (27°C) *(37)*.

STUDIES OF POSTISCHEMIC HYPOTHERMIA IN GLOBAL ISCHEMIA

The salutary influence of mild to moderate degrees of intraischemic hypothermia in models of global ischemia raised the clinically relevant issue of whether *postischemic* cooling to the same degree would also

---

Fig. 1. *(previous page)* Paraffin-embedded coronal brain sections stained with hematoxylin and eosin from normothermic–ischemic (a, b) and hypothermic–ischemic (c, d) rats. (a) Two months after 12.5 min of normothermic (37°C) global ischemia, severe necrosis of CA1 hippocampus is evident (×120). (b) Higher magnification of injured CA1 sector illustrates only two viable neurons *(arrowheads)* among reactive astrocytes and microglia (×1100). (c) In contrast to the normothermic results, a relatively intact CA1 sector is present in a rat that had undergone hypothermic (30°C) global ischemia (×120). (d) Higher magnification of CA1 demonstrates many viable neurons containing a distinct nucleus and nucleolus (×1100). [Reproduced with permission from Green E. J., et al. (1992) *Brain Research* **580,** 197–204. Elsevier Science Publishers, B. V.]

protect. Several questions arose: How quickly must hypothermia be initiated after ischemia to be neuroprotective? For how long and to what depth should it be administered? Is the resulting neuroprotection temporary or permanent? Using a model of 10-min normothermic global forebrain ischemia by the two-vessel occlusion model, we compared the neuropathological outcome when cranial cooling to 30°C was begun at either 5 or 30 min following the ischemic insult, and was maintained for 3 h *(38)*. In these initial studies, in which only a 3-d survival was permitted, 50% protection of hippocampal CA1 pyramidal neurons was achieved when cooling was begun at 5 min postischemia, but cooling was ineffective if deferred until 30 min. Other workers showed that cooling to 34°C for 2 h following normothermic ischemia provided partial histological protection of hippocampal neurons if the insult was only 8 min in duration but failed to protect if the ischemic insult lasted 12 min *(30,39)*. In a gerbil study of 5-min global ischemia at 38°C (a severe insult), followed by prompt temperature reduction to 33°C for 1 h or to 23°C for 2 h, hippocampal CA1 injury was extensive despite the cooling *(40)*. In other studies examining the effect of postischemic cooling duration, 6 h of immediate postischemic hypothermia conferred histological protection whereas a 1-h cooling period did not *(41)*. Postischemic hypothermia of approx 33°C begun at 2 h postischemia conferred hippocampal protection if continued for 5 h *(42)*.

A crucial, clinically relevant issue is whether postischemic cooling confers *permanent* neuroprotection. Certain observations described above suggested that this might not be the case *(40)*. By contrast, our studies of *intraischemic* hypothermia had shown enduring neuroprotection out to 2 mo (**Fig. 1**) *(38,43)*. This issue was tested in a study in which rats were subjected to 10 min of normothermic ischemia followed by a 3-h period of cranial hypothermia (30°C) and survival for either 3 d, 7 d, or 2 mo *(44)*. In hypothermic animals with 3-d survival, significant protection of CA1 pyramidal neurons was observed, but this protective effect declined in rats surviving for 7 d and was lost in rats surviving for 2 mo. This result contrasted with the permanent protection seen at 2 mo in a similar insult under conditions of intraischemic hypothermia. This study thus indicated that, in contrast to intraischemic cooling, postischemic hypothermia is capable of *delaying* the onset of ischemic cell change but may not permanently protect, and it emphasized the importance of chronic survival studies in assessing neuroprotection. These results also raised the possibility that the cellular and molecular mechanisms of intra- vs postischemic cooling might differ from one another.

The delay in onset of ischemic cell change with postischemic cooling raised the possibility that this therapy might, in fact, extend the therapeutic window for intervention with other (e.g., pharmacological) neuroprotectants. This proved to be the case in a study in which rats receiving 10-min of global ischemia followed by 3-h postischemic cooling to 30°C were subsequently treated with the noncompetitive *N*-methyl-D-aspartate (NMDA) antagonist dizocilpine administered on postischemic d 3, 5, and 7. Partial permanent hippocampal neuroprotection resulted from the combined therapy *(45)*. Similarly, postischemic hypothermia combined with delayed administration of *n-tert*-butyl-α-phenylnitrone (PBN), a free radical spin-trap agent, led to long-term cognitive improvement *(46)*. In rats with 12.5 min of normothermic ischemia, 4 h of postischemic hypothermia (33–34°C) alone failed to protect the CA1 hippocampus 2 mo later, whereas the combination of hypothermia plus interleukin-10 administration conferred long-lasting partial protection *(47)*. The potential clinical implications of these findings are obvious.

Studies in other laboratories have substantiated that more prolonged periods of postischemic cooling alone do, in fact, confer a more permanent degree of neuroprotection. In gerbil studies with 30-d survival, when cooling to 32°C was instituted for 12 h beginning 1 h after a global ischemic insult, substantially reduced CA1 necrosis resulted when the insult was mild (3-min insult), but this effect was only partial when a 5-min insult had been used *(48)*. When the cooling period was prolonged to 24 h, the 5-min ischemic animals exhibited much greater degrees of neuroprotection at 30 d. A subsequent study extended the survival time to 6 mo and showed enduring neuroprotection with prolonged postischemic cooling *(49)*. A still more recent study explored an analogous paradigm in rats with 10-min of severe forebrain ischemia exposed to a 48-h period of mild hypothermia starting 6 h after the insult. A 28-d survival was permitted. Robust, enduring CA1 protection was obtained *(50)*. Postischemic hypothermia is considered in detail elsewhere in this volume, and the subject has been recently reviewed extensively *(51)*.

An important implication of the aforementioned findings is the possibility that neuroprotective effects might be falsely ascribed to pharmacological agents that acted by inadvertently producing hypothermia.

This proved to be the case for the NMDA antagonist dizocilpine (MK-801), which had initially been reported to be highly neuro-protective in some (but not all) global ischemia studies *(52,53)*. Further investigation revealed that this neuroprotective effect was associated with prolonged hypothermia *(54)*, which, when prevented, abrogated the "protective" effect of the drug. It is highly likely that the putative neuroprotective effect ascribed to other pharmacological agents (e.g., barbiturates) may, in retrospect, also have been explicable on the basis of unnoticed hypothermia.

THE OBVERSE OF HYPOTHERMIA: THE DELETERIOUS EFFECT OF HYPERTHERMIA

Ten years ago, it was observed in a model of 5-min global ischemia in gerbils that the expected severe hippocampal neuronal loss could be markedly attenuated by prolonging the period of halothane anesthesia, which blunted the mild postischemic hyperthermia (approx 1.5°C) that would otherwise occur *(55)*. This effect was not specific to halothane but rather could be duplicated by warming the head by a similar amount in its absence. This study established the marked sensitivity of the postischemic brain to even mild hyperthermia.

Early in our studies of hypothermia, we observed that warming the brain to 39°C during a 20-min global ischemic insult accentuated ischemic changes in cortex, hippocampus, and subcortical structures *(21)*. A careful study comparing the sequelae of 20-min global ischemia in rats under conditions of intraischemic temperatures of either 37°C or 39°C revealed both an acceleration and marked accentuation of injury in the hyperthermic group, in which evidence of severe neuronal injury was present at even 1-d survival *(21,56)*. Severe ischemic changes were present in striatum and hippocampus; laminar necrosis was seen in the cortex; focal thalamic infarction occurred, and widespread ischemic changes involved other structures. This deleterious effect of hyperther-mia was confirmed in the rat *(28)* and gerbil *(57)*.

We subsequently used a rat model of 5- or 7-min global ischemia by two-vessel occlusion to study whether delayed hyperthermia instituted after an ischemic insult would exacerbate injury. Twenty-four hours after ischemia, rats of one group were exposed to elevated ambient temperature so as to raise rectal temperature to 39–40°C for 3 h *(58)*. Following an 8-d survival, histopathological examination in rats with 7-min ischemia revealed that delayed hyperthermia led to an approximately 2.6-fold increase in numbers of ischemic neurons in the hippocampal CA1 sector; a similar but nonsignificant trend was seen in the 5-min ischemic group *(58)*. A comparable study was conducted in a model of 60-min transient focal ischemia—an insult ordinarily giving rise to a small subcortical infarction. When body temperature was elevated to 40°C for 3 h 1 d after middle cerebral artery occlusion, infarct volume was dramatically increased *(59)*.

Interestingly, these observations appear to have important clinical relevance. Direct monitoring of intracranial temperature in neurosurgical patients with head injury and other conditions has revealed that brain temperatures commonly exceed rectal temperatures and, in the injured brain, this gradient may be as high as 2.5°C *(60)*. Thus, it might be expected that systemic fever of a given degree would result in even greater elevations of brain temperature in the injured brain. Similarly, during rewarming following hypothermic cardiac surgery, cerebral temperature (as reflected in cerebral venous temperature) may quickly rise to 39°C or higher *(61)*. In patients with acute stroke, several studies have now shown a correlation between elevated temperature and poor outcome *(62,63)*. Fever of 38°C or above proved to be an independent factor predicting worse prognosis and higher mortality *(62)*. A 1°C difference in body temperature increased the relative risk of poor outcome by 2.2-fold *(63)*. In 260 patients with acute hemispheric ischemic stroke in whom body temperature was recorded every 2 h, axillary temperature >37.5°C during the first 24 h after stroke onset was highly correlated to larger infarct volumes at 3 mo *(64)*.

Hyperthermia appears to act through several mechanisms to worsen cerebral ischemia. Intraischemic hyperthermia accentuates and prolongs the release of extracellular glutamate; it also accentuates the release of γ-aminobutyric acid and glycine and markedly increases the so-called "excitotoxic index"—a composite measure of neurotransmitter release *(65,66)*. Comparable results were observed in a model of focal ischemia *(67)*. In patients with acute stroke, cerebrospinal fluid (CSF) concentrations of glutamate and glycine correlated with increased body temperature, suggesting that excitotoxic mechanisms may contribute to the hyperthermia-associated worsening *(68)*.

Postischemic oxygen radical production is also accentuated by hyperthermia. Microdialysis studies sampling the brain's extracellular fluid for a signal of hydroxyl radical production have revealed two- to threefold elevations after normothermic global ischemia, but four- to fivefold elevations after mildly hyperthermic (39°C) ischemia *(69,70)*. Ischemia-induced blood–brain barrier (BBB) opening is also highly sensitive to brain temperature. Following mild intraischemic hyperthermia (39°C), marked accentuation of BBB breakdown has been described *(71,72)*. Magnetic resonance spectroscopy studies have revealed enhanced intracellular acidosis and impaired recovery of cerebral energy metabolites in cats with global cerebral ischemia under hyperthermic conditions *(73)*. Similar findings were obtained by direct assay of energy metabolites *(74)*.

Hyperthermia affects a number of intracellular processes. For example, temperatures of 39°C during ischemia accentuate the inhibition of calcium/calmodulin-dependent protein kinase II induced by brief global ischemia *(57)*. Patterns of protein kinase C alterations induced by global ischemia are also significantly influenced by hyperthermia *(75)*. Mild intraischemic hyperthermia during global ischemia in gerbils aggravated the decreases in calmodulin and microtubule-associated protein 2 (MAP2) immunoreactivities in hippocampus *(76)*.

These observations (as well as corroborative evidence in focal ischemia, not reviewed here) have led us to offer the strong recommendation that *body temperature be maintained in a safe normothermic range (e.g., 36.7–37°C) for at least the first several days after the onset of acute stroke or head injury*, and that caution should be taken to avoid rewarming following hypothermic cardiopulmonary bypass *(77)*.

MECHANISMS
OF HYPOTHERMIC NEUROPROTECTION

Cerebral Blood Flow and Metabolism

The effect of hypothermia on cerebral perfusion appears to vary according to the method of cooling (systemic vs local) and the level of temperature reduction. Both increases and decreases of cerebral blood flow (CBF) have been reported. During a global ischemic insult itself, direct measurements have shown that the degree of CBF reduction during ischemia is unaffected by the intraischemic temperature level *(21,78)*. In like manner, assays of brain energy metabolites following global ischemia have shown that the magnitudes of high-energy phosphate depletion and lactate elevation are similar, irrespective of intraischemic temperature over the range of 30–39°C *(74)*. Although intraischemic hypothermia does not appear to act via an alteration of energy metabolite levels, other studies suggest that the *initial* rate of

ATP depletion during global ischemia is retarded by mild hypothermia *(79–81)*. This slowing of the rate of ATP depletion may contribute significantly to the protective effect of hypothermia. Conflicting data appear in the literature as to whether hypothermia alters cerebral lactate accumulation, with both negative findings *(82)* and reduced acidosis *(83)* being reported. Magnetic resonance spectroscopy studies in rats with forebrain ischemia have shown that the postischemic intracellular alkalosis present with normothermia is abolished in hypothermic animals *(84)*. In an extensive study of regional brain energy metabolites by direct sampling following 20-min global ischemia at intraischemic cranial temperatures of 30°C, 37°C, or 39°C *(74)*, somewhat less complete recovery of ATP levels and the sum of adenylates was observed in the hyperthermic group.

Studies assessing local cerebral glucose utilization (lCMRglu) and blood flow (lCBF) in the postischemic state in rats with 20-min global ischemia have shown significantly greater recovery of lCMRglu throughout cortical and subcortical structures of rats with intraischemic hypothermia compared to normothermic animals *(85)*. Autoradiographic studies have also revealed improved metabolic activation in response to peripheral stimuli following global ischemia conducted under hypothermic compared to normothermic circumstances *(86)*.

Neurotransmitter Release

A major mechanism of ischemic injury is thought to involve the release and extracellular accumulation of excitatory amino acids in ischemia, leading to excessive activation of postsynaptic glutamate receptors, increases in intracellular free calcium ion concentration, and a subsequent cascade of complex events leading to cell death *(87–89)*. Multiple neurotransmitters and neuromodulators are massively released in ischemia, including dopamine, norepinephrine, serotonin, and others *(90–92)*. Hypothermic temperatures tend to inhibit the biosynthesis, release, and/or reuptake of these various neurotransmitters *(93,94)*. Our laboratory has shown that in rats with 20-min global ischemia by two-vessel occlusion, mild intraischemic hypothermia markedly diminishes the extent of glutamate release in the striatum *(78)*. During normothermia, there is a sevenfold surge of glutamate above baseline levels; this is completely inhibited by brain temperature reductions to 33°C or 30°C *(78,90,95)*. Similarly, the 500-fold release of dopamine in normothermic ischemia is attenuated by approximately 60% at hypothermic temperatures of 33°C or 30°C. Microdialysis studies in other laboratories have confirmed these findings *(96)*. In rabbits with 10-min global ischemia, marked attenuations of glutamate, aspartate, and glycine release were reported at epidural temperature reductions of 20°C *(97)*. Other studies of transient global ischemia in hypothermic rabbits have confirmed profoundly reduced levels of hippocampal glutamate and glycine *(98,99)*. The hypothermic inhibition of glutamate increase has been demonstrated also under conditions of ischemia complicated by hyperglycemia *(100)*. By means of a real-time method for monitoring extracellular glutamate levels, it was shown that hypothermia appears to enhance postischemic glutamate reuptake *(101)*.

The excitotoxic index was developed by our group as a composite descriptor of excitatory/inhibitory amino acid neurotransmitter balance as measured by microdialysis in the brain's extracellular space *(66,102)*. This index is defined as:

$$\text{Excitotoxic index} = [\text{glutamate}] \times [\text{glycine}]/[\text{GABA}]$$

Our group was able to show that 12.5 min of normothermic global ischemia led to significant, 7- to 12-fold increases in the striatal excitotoxic index that persisted for 3–4 h. By contrast, animals with postischemic hypothermia (30°C for 3 h) showed no changes in the excitotoxic index during recirculation *(103)*.

The preceding observations are obviously relevant to the neuroprotective effect of *intraischemic* hypothermia. Late increases in extracellular glutamate and aspartate levels have also been reported after ischemia *(104)* and following multiple ischemic insults *(105)*. It is possible that prolonged postischemic hypothermia may affect these late processes, although this has not been established.

Intracellular Messengers and Mediators

Hypothermia has been shown to affect a variety of intracellular mediators, although an integrated synthesis has not yet emerged. Studies in our laboratory have shown that inositol 1,4,5-trisphosphate (IP$_3$) decreases significantly in cortex and subcortical structures during normothermic global ischemia, but these declines are partially mitigated by intraischemic hypothermia *(106)*. Protein kinase C (PKC) is a calcium-dependent enzyme activated by diacylglycerol and produced in the course of inositol phospholipid hydrolysis. Its activation involves a translocation from cytosol to the cell membrane. Translocation and inhibition of PKC occur during ischemia *(107,108)*. One study reported an absence of PKC translocation and a lack of its inhibition with intraischemic hypothermia *(109)*. In another study, intraischemic temperature highly influenced PKC activity during recirculation *(75)*. In normothermic rats, significantly reduced PKC activity was observed at all recirculation time points, but in the hypothermic group normal PKC levels were observed during ischemia and reperfusion. Conversely, *hyperthermia* significantly decreased PKC activity in both controls and ischemic animals *(75)*. Similar findings were obtained in a global forebrain ischemia model in which mild hypothermia applied intraischemically and during reperfusion (60 min) inhibited translocation of PKC-α, β, γ isoforms as well as fodrin proteolysis *(110)*.

Calcium/calmodulin-dependent protein kinase II (CaM kinase II) is a mediator of synaptic and cytoskeletal function as well as neurotransmitter release. The reduced CaM kinase II activity observed following normothermic ischemia is not seen under conditions of intraischemic hypothermia *(57,110)*. Ubiquitin, a small protein involved in the catabolism of other abnormal proteins, is decreased following ischemia; this may lead to an accumulation of abnormal proteins that affect cell function. Intraischemic hypothermia induces a significant restitution of ubiquitin compared to the normothermic condition *(111)*.

BBB Breakdown

The extent to which the BBB is influenced by ischemia is highly temperature dependent. Early BBB breakdown to protein tracers is demonstrable after normothermic global ischemia but is suppressed by mild to moderate hypothermia and is greatly accentuated by intraischemic hyperthermia *(71,112)*. Similarly, postischemic edema following global ischemia is reduced by moderate hypothermia *(113)*.

Reactive Oxygen Species

Oxygen free radicals are elaborated during ischemia and reperfusion and have been strongly implicated in the pathophysiology of ischemic brain injury *(114)*. These reactions may lead to oxidative injury to cellular lipids, proteins, and nucleic acids. Evidence for free radical elaboration in ischemia is obtainable by means of a microdialysis method in which administered salicylate is converted, in the presence of hydroxyl radical, to dihydroxybenzoic acid (DHBA) species—stable adducts detectable by chromatographic methods. A study from our laboratory of

20-min global ischemia documented substantial early elevations of the DHBA signal from striatum following 20 min of normothermic global ischemia *(69)*. These elevations were strikingly exaggerated following hyperthermic (39°C) ischemia and, conversely, were completely attenuated following hypothermic (30°C) ischemia of similar duration.

Inflammatory mechanisms involving polymorphonuclear leukocytes may, in part, mediate radical-induced pathology in ischemia. In focal ischemia, intraischemic hypothermia was shown to attenuate neutrophil infiltration *(115)*.

Gene Expression and Protein Synthesis

A generalized depression of protein synthesis occurs following global ischemia and may affect the translation of messages such as those for immediate early genes, which are rapidly transcribed after ischemia. Moderate hypothermia (30°C) during ischemia reverses the postischemic inhibition of protein synthesis *(116)*. Detailed studies *(117)* suggest that intraischemic hypothermia affects transcriptional events in a temporally and spatially complex fashion. Hypothermia appears to enhance the expression of certain immediate early genes following ischemia; this may be consistent with the promotion of cell survival. In a model of 10-min forebrain ischemia in the gerbil, intraischemic hypothermia (30°C) hastened the time course of expression of the immediate early genes c-*fos* and *fos*-B in hippocampal regions, again suggesting a possible recovery-associated mechanism *(118)*.

Similarly, following 10 min of forebrain ischemia, mild hypothermia applied for 3 h attenuated apoptotic death in hippocampal neurons 72 h postinsult *(119)*. The neuroprotection appeared to be correlated with increased expression of Bcl-2, an antiapoptotic protein.

While moderate *intra*ischemic hypothermia (33°C) failed to increase the expression of mRNAs for the neurotrophins nerve growth factor (NGF), brain-derived neurotrophic factor (BDNF), neurotrophin-3 (NT3), or TrkB in ischemia-sensitive hippocampal subregions, hypothermia did induce neurotrophin mRNA alterations in the ischemia-resistant dentate gyrus; it was speculated that this might confer protection *(120)*. In contrast, *post*ischemic hypothermia (33°C) potentiated the increase in BDNF at 24 h postcardiac arrest (8-min duration) and increased tissue levels of and tyrosine phosphorylation of TrkB *(121)*. In this study it was suggested that increased activation of BDNF signaling could be a possible mechanism by which mild hypothermia reduces neuronal injury after global cerebral ischemia.

CONCLUSIONS

Investigations from laboratories throughout the world accrued over the past dozen years have established with certitude the neuroprotective influence of mild to moderate degrees of brain hypothermia in the setting of global (and focal) cerebral ischemia. Conversely, mild hyperthermia has emerged as an important factor exacerbating ischemic brain injury. The avoidance of fever in patients with acute brain injury should now be part of routine clinical practice. Randomized trials of therapeutic hypothermia will be required to establish efficacy in patients with brain ischemia; in the modern intensive care setting, they are eminently feasible.

ACKNOWLEDGMENTS

This work was supported by NIH Program Project Grant NS 05820.

REFERENCES

1. Ginsberg M.D., Sternau L. L., Globus M. Y., Dietrich W. D., and Busto R. (1992) Therapeutic modulation of brain temperature: relevance to ischemic brain injury. *Cerebrovasc. Brain Metab. Rev.* **4,** 189–225.
2. Smith L. W. and Fay T. (1939) Temperature factors in cancer and embryonal cell growth. *JAMA* **113,** 653–660.
3. Fay T. (1943) Observations on generalized refrigeration in cases of severe cerebral trauma. *Assoc. Res. Nerv. Ment. Dis. Proc.* **24,** 611–619.
4. Fay T. and Smith G. W. (1941) Observations on reflex responses during prolonged periods of human refrigeration. *Arch. Neurol. Psychiatry* **45,** 215–222.
5. Berger R. L. (1990) Nazi science—the Dachau hypothermia experiments. *N. Engl. J. Med.* **322,** 1435–1446.
6. Sealy W. C., Brown I. J., and Young W. J. (1958) A report on the use of both extracorporeal circulation and hypothermia for open heart surgery. *Ann. Surg.* **147,** 603–613.
7. Botterell E. H., Lougheed W. M., Scott J. W., and Vandewater S. L. (1956) Hypothermia, and interruption of carotid, or carotid and vertebral circulation, in the surgical management of intracranial aneurysms. *J. Neurosurg.* **13,** 1–42.
8. Spetzler R. F., Hadley M. N., Rigamonti D., et al. (1988) Aneurysms of the basilar artery treated with circulatory arrest, hypothermia, and barbiturate cerebral protection. *J. Neurosurg.* **68,** 868–879.
9. Weinrauch V., Safar P., Tisherman S., Kuboyama K., and Radovsky A. (1992) Beneficial effect of mild hypothermia and detrimental effect of deep hypothermia after cardiac arrest in dogs. *Stroke* **23,** 1454–1462.
10. Busto R. and Ginsberg M. D. (1998) The influence of altered brain temperature in cerebral ischemia. In *Cerebrovascular Disease: Pathophysiology, Diagnosis and Management* (Ginsberg M. D. and Bogousslavsky, J., eds.), Blackwell Science, Malden, pp. 287–307.

11. Rosomoff H. L. and Holaday D. A. (1954) Cerebral blood flow and cerebral oxygen consumption during hypothermia. *Am. J. Physiol.* **179,** 85–88.
12. Hagerdal M., Harp J., Nilsson L., and Siesjo B. K. (1975) The effect of induced hypothermia upon oxygen consumption in the rat brain. *J. Neurochem.* **24,** 311–316.
13. Rosomoff H. L. (1957) Hypothermia and cerebral vascular lesions. II. Experimental middle cerebral artery interruption followed by induction of hypothermia. *AMA Arch. Neurol. Psychiatry* **78,** 454–464.
14. Rosomoff H. L. (1959) Experimental brain injury during hypothermia. *J. Neurosurg.* **16,** 177–187.
15. Connoly J. E., Boyd R. J., and Calvin J. W. (1962) The protective effect of hypothermia in cerebral ischemia: experimental and clinical application by selective brain cooling in the human. *Surgery* **52,** 15–24.
16. Senning A. and Olsson P. I. (1956) Changes in vascular tonus during cerebral and regional hypothermia. *Acta Chir. Scand.* **112,** 209–219.
17. White R. J., Massopust L. A., Jr., Wolin L. R., Taslitz N., and Yashon D. (1969) Profound selective cooling and ischaemia of primate brain without pump or oxygenator. *Br. J. Surg.* **56,** 630–631.
18. Hirsch H. and Müller H. A. (1962) Funktionelle und histologische Veränderungen des Kaninchengehirns nach kompletter Gehirnischämie. *Pflug. Arch.* **275,** 277–291.
19. Berntman L., Welsh F. A., and Harp J. R. (1981) Cerebral protective effect of low-grade hypothermia. *Anesthesiology* **55,** 495–498.
20. Vibulsresth S., Dietrich W. D., Busto R., and Ginsberg M. D. (1987) Failure of nimodipine to prevent ischemic neuronal damage in rats. *Stroke* **18,** 210–216.
21. Busto R., Dietrich W. D., Globus M. Y., Valdes I., Scheinberg P., and Ginsberg M. D. (1987) Small differences in intraischemic brain temperature critically determine the extent of ischemic neuronal injury. *J. Cereb. Blood Flow Metab.* **7,** 729–738.
22. Smith M. L., Auer R. N., and Siesjö B. K. (1984) The density and distribution of ischemic brain injury in the rat following 2–10 min of forebrain ischemia. *Acta Neuropathol (Berl.)* **64,** 319–322.
23. Pulsinelli W. A. and Brierley J. B. (1979) A new model of bilateral hemispheric ischemia in the unanesthetized rat. *Stroke* **10,** 267–272.
24. Thornhill J. and Asselin J. (1999) The effect of head cooling on the physiological responses and resultant neural damage to global hemispheric hypoxic ischemia in prostaglandin E2 treated rats. *Brain Res.* **825,** 36–45.
25. Nurse S. and Corbett D. (1994) Direct measurement of brain temperature during and after intraischemic hypothermia: correlation with behavioral, physiological, and histological endpoints. *J. Neurosci.* **14,** 7726–7734.
26. Clifton G. L., Taft W. C., Blair R. E., Choi S. C., and DeLorenzo R. J. (1989) Conditions for pharmacologic evaluation in the gerbil model of forebrain ischemia. *Stroke* **20,** 1545–1552.
27. Minamisawa H., Nordström C. H., Smith M. L., and Siesjö B. K. (1990) The influence of mild body and brain hypothermia on ischemic brain damage. *J. Cereb. Blood Flow Metab.* **10,** 365–374.
28. Minamisawa H., Smith M. L., and Siesjö B. K. (1990) The effect of mild hyperthermia and hypothermia on brain damage following 5, 10, and 15 minutes of forebrain ischemia. *Ann. Neurol.* **28,** 26–33.

29. Kuluz J. W., Gregory G. A., Yu A. C., and Chang Y. (1992) Selective brain cooling during and after prolonged global ischemia reduces cortical damage in rats. *Stroke* **23,** 1792–1796.

30. Chopp M., Chen H., Dereski M. O., and Garcia J. H. (1991) Mild hypothermic intervention after graded ischemic stress in rats. *Stroke* **22,** 37–43.

31. Freund T. F., Buzsaki G., Leon A., and Somogyi P. (1990) Hippocampal cell death following ischemia: effects of brain temperature and anesthesia. *Exp. Neurol.* **108,** 251–260.

32. Lundgren J., Smith M. L., and Siesjö B. K. (1991) Influence of moderate hypothermia on ischemic brain damage incurred under hyperglycemic conditions. *Exp. Brain Res.* **84,** 91–101.

33. Leonov Y., Sterz F., Safar P., et al. (1990) Mild cerebral hypothermia during and after cardiac arrest improves neurologic outcome in dogs. *J. Cereb. Blood Flow Metab.* **10,** 57–70.

34. Kuboyama K., Safar P., Radovsky A., Tisherman S. A., Stezoski S. W., and Alexander H. (1993) Delay in cooling negates the beneficial effect of mild resuscitative cerebral hypothermia after cardiac arrest in dogs: a prospective, randomized study. *Crit. Care Med.* **21,** 1348–1358.

35. Wass C. T., Lanier W. L., Hofer R. E., Scheithauer B. W., and Andrews A. G. (1995) Temperature changes of > or = 1 degree C alter functional neurologic outcome and histopathology in a canine model of complete cerebral ischemia. *Anesthesiology* **83,** 325–335.

36. Horn M., Schlote W., and Henrich H. A. (1991) Global cerebral ischemia and subsequent selective hypothermia. A neuropathological and morphometrical study on ischemic neuronal damage in cat. *Acta Neuropathol. (Berl.)* **81,** 443–449.

37. Laursen H., Waaben J., Gefke K., Husum B., Andersen L. I., and Sorensen H. R. (1989) Brain histology, blood-brain barrier and brain water after normothermic and hypothermic cardiopulmonary bypass in pigs. *Eur. J. Cardiothorac. Surg.* **3,** 539–543.

38. Busto R., Dietrich W. D., Globus M. Y., and Ginsberg M. D. (1989) Postischemic moderate hypothermia inhibits CA1 hippocampal ischemic neuronal injury. *Neurosci. Lett.* **101,** 299–304.

39. Chen H., Chopp M., Vande Linde A. M., Dereski M. O., Garcia J. H., and Welch K. M. (1992) The effects of post-ischemic hypothermia on the neuronal injury and brain metabolism after forebrain ischemia in the rat. *J. Neurol. Sci.* **107,** 191–198.

40. Welsh F. A. and Harris V. A. (1991) Postischemic hypothermia fails to reduce ischemic injury in gerbil hippocampus. *J. Cereb. Blood Flow Metab.* **11,** 617–620.

41. Carroll M. and Beek O. (1992) Protection against hippocampal CA1 cell loss by post-ischemic hypothermia is dependent on delay of initiation and duration. *Metab. Brain Dis.* **7,** 45–50.

42. Coimbra C. and Wieloch T. (1994) Moderate hypothermia mitigates neuronal damage in the rat brain when initiated several hours following transient cerebral ischemia. *Acta Neuropathol.* **87,** 325–331.

43. Green E. J., Dietrich W. D., van Dijk F., et al. (1992) Protective effects of brain hypothermia on behavior and histopathology following global cerebral ischemia in rats. *Brain Res.* **580,** 197–204.

44. Dietrich W. D., Busto R., Alonso O., Globus M. Y., and Ginsberg M. D. (1993) Intraischemic but not postischemic brain hypothermia protects chronically following global forebrain ischemia in rats. *J. Cereb. Blood Flow Metab.* **13,** 541–549.

45. Dietrich W. D., Lin B., Globus M. Y., Green E. J., Ginsberg M. D., and Busto R. (1995) Effect of delayed MK-801 (dizocilpine) treatment with or without immediate postischemic hypothermia on chronic neuronal survival after global forebrain ischemia in rats. *J. Cerebr. Blood Flow Metab.* **15,** 960–968.
46. Pazos A. J., Green E. J., Busto R., et al. (1999) Effects of combined postischemic hypothermia and delayed *N*-tert-butyl-alpha-pheylnitrone (PBN) administration on histopathological and behavioral deficits associated with transient global ischemia in rats. *Brain Res.* **846,** 186–195.
47. Dietrich W. D., Busto R., and Bethea J. R. (1999) Postischemic hypothermia and IL-10 treatment provide long-lasting neuroprotection of CA1 hippocampus following transient global ischemia in rats. *Exp. Neurol.* **158,** 444–450.
48. Colbourne F. and Corbett D. (1994) Delayed and prolonged post-ischemic hypothermia is neuroprotective in the gerbil. *Brain Res.* **654,** 265–272.
49. Colbourne F. and Corbett D. (1995) Delayed postischemic hypothermia: a six month survival study using behavioral and histological assessments of neuroprotection. *J. Neurosci.* **15,** 7250–7260.
50. Colbourne F., Li H., and Buchan A. M. (1999) Indefatigable CA1 sector neuroprotection with mild hypothermia induced 6 hours after severe forebrain ischemia in rats. *J. Cereb. Blood Flow Metab.* **19,** 742–749.
51. Colbourne F., Sutherland G., and Corbett D. (1997) Postischemic hypothermia. A critical appraisal with implications for clinical treatment. *Mol. Neurobiol.* **14,** 171–201.
52. Gill R., Foster A. C., and Woodruff G. N. (1988) MK-801 is neuroprotective in gerbils when administered during the post-ischaemic period. *Neuroscience* **25,** 847–855.
53. Buchan A. M. (1990) Do NMDA antagonists protect against cerebral ischemia: are clinical trials warranted? *Cerebrovasc. Brain Metab. Rev.* **2,** 1–26.
54. Buchan A. and Pulsinelli W. A. (1990) Hypothermia but not the N-methyl-D-aspartate antagonist, MK-801, attenuates neuronal damage in gerbils subjected to transient global ischemia. *J. Neurosci.* **10,** 311–316.
55. Kuroiwa T., Bonnekoh P., and Hossmann K. A. (1990) Prevention of postischemic hyperthermia prevents ischemic injury of CA1 neurons in gerbils. *J. Cereb. Blood Flow Metab.* **10,** 550–556.
56. Dietrich W. D., Busto R., Valdes I., and Loor Y. (1990) Effects of normothermic versus mild hyperthermic forebrain ischemia in rats. *Stroke* **21,** 1318–1325.
57. Churn S. B., Taft W. C., Billingsley M. S., Blair R. E., and DeLorenzo R. J. (1990) Temperature modulation of ischemic neuronal death and inhibition of calcium/calmodulin-dependent protein kinase II in gerbils. *Stroke* **21,** 1715–1721.
58. Baena R. C., Busto R., Dietrich W. D., Globus M. Y., and Ginsberg M. D. (1997) Hyperthermia delayed by 24 hours aggravates neuronal damage in rat hippocampus following global ischemia. *Neurology* **48,** 768–773.
59. Kim Y., Truettner J., Zhao W., Busto R., and Ginsberg M. D. (1998) The influence of delayed postischemic hyperthermia following transient focal ischemia: alterations of gene expression. *J. Neurol. Sci.* **159,** 1–10.
60. Mellergard P. and Nordstrom C. H. (1991) Intracerebral temperature in neurosurgical patients. *Neurosurgery* **28,** 709–713.
61. Cook D. J., Orszulak T. A., Daly R. C., and Buda D. A. (1996) Cerebral hyperthermia during cardiopulmonary bypass in adults. *J. Thorac. Cardiovasc. Surg.* **111,** 268–269.

62. Azzimondi G., Bassein L., Nonino F., et al. (1995) Fever in acute stroke worsens prognosis. A prospective study. *Stroke* **26**, 2040–2043.
63. Reith J., Jorgensen H. S., Pedersen P. M., et al. (1996) Body temperature in acute stroke: relation to stroke severity, infarct size, mortality, and outcome. *Lancet* **347**, 422–425.
64. Castillo J., Davalos A., Marrugat J., and Noya M. (1998) Timing for fever-related brain damage in acute ischemic stroke. *Stroke* **29**, 2455–2460.
65. Sternau L. L., Globus M. Y., Dietrich W. D., Martinez E., Busto R., and Ginsberg M. D. (1992) Ischemia-induced neurotransmitter release: effects of mild intraischemic hyperthermia. In *The Role of Neurotransmitters in Brain Injury* (Globus M. Y. and Dietrich W. D., eds.), Plenum Press, New York, pp. 33–38.
66. Globus M. Y., Ginsberg M. D., and Busto R. (1991) Excitotoxic index—a biochemical marker of selective vulnerability. *Neurosci. Lett.* **127**, 39–42.
67. Takagi K., Ginsberg M. D., Globus M. Y., Martinez E., and Busto R. (1994) Effect of hyperthermia on glutamate release in ischemic penumbra after middle cerebral artery occlusion in rats. *Am. J. Physiol.* **267**, H1770–1776.
68. Castillo J., Davalos A., and Noya M. (1999) Aggravation of acute ischemic stroke by hyperthermia is related to an excitotoxic mechanism. *Cerebrovasc. Dis.* **9**, 22–27.
69. Globus M. Y., Busto R., Lin B., Schnippering H., and Ginsberg M. D. (1995) Detection of free radical activity during transient global ischemia and recirculation: effects of intraischemic brain temperature modulation. *J. Neurochem.* **65**, 1250–1256.
70. Kil H. Y., Zhang J., and Piantadosi C. A. (1996) Brain temperature alters hydroxyl radical production during cerebral ischemia/reperfusion in rats. *J. Cereb. Blood Flow Metab.* **16**, 100–106.
71. Dietrich W. D., Busto R., Halley M., and Valdes I. (1990) The importance of brain temperature in alterations of the blood-brain barrier following cerebral ischemia. *J. Neuropathol. Exp. Neurol.* **49**, 486–497.
72. Dietrich W. D., Halley M., Valdes I., and Busto R. (1991) Interrelationships between increased vascular permeability and acute neuronal damage following temperature-controlled brain ischemia in rats. *Acta Neuropathol.* **81**, 615–625.
73. Chopp M., Welch K. M., Tidwell C. D., Knight R., and Helpern J. A. (1988) Effect of mild hyperthermia on recovery of metabolic function after global cerebral ischemia in cats. *Stroke* **19**, 1521–1525.
74. Ginsberg M. D., Busto R., Martinez E., Globus M. Y., Valdes I., and Loor Y. (1992) The effects of cerebral ischemia on energy metabolism. In *Drug Research Related to Neuroactive Amino Acids—Alfred Benzon Symposium 32* (Schousboe A., Diemer N. H., and Kofod H., eds.), Munksgaard, Copenhagen, pp. 207–224.
75. Busto R., Globus M. Y., Neary J. T., and Ginsberg M. D. (1994) Regional alterations of protein kinase C activity following transient cerebral ischemia: effects of intraischemic brain temperature modulation. *J. Neurochem.* **63**, 1095–1103.
76. Eguchi Y., Yamashita K., Iwamoto T., and Ito H. (1997) Effects of brain temperature on calmodulin and microtubule-associated protein 2 immunoreactivity in the gerbil hippocampus following transient forebrain ischemia. *J. Neurotrauma* **14**, 109–118.
77. Ginsberg M. D. and Busto R. (1998) Combating hyperthermia in acute stroke: a significant clinical concern. *Stroke* **29**, 529–534.

78. Busto R., Globus M. Y., Dietrich W. D., Martinez E., Valdes I., and Ginsberg M. D. (1989) Effect of mild hypothermia on ischemia-induced release of neurotransmitters and free fatty acids in rat brain. *Stroke* **20,** 904–910.

79. Kramer R. S., Sanders A. P., Lesage A. M., Woodhall B., and Sealy W. C. (1968) The effect profound hypothermia on preservation of cerebral ATP content during circulatory arrest. *J. Thorac. Cardiovasc. Surg.* **56,** 699–709.

80. Michenfelder J. D. and Theye R. A. (1970) The effects of anesthesia and hypothermia on canine cerebral ATP and lactate during anoxia produced by decapitation. *Anesthesiology* **33,** 430–439.

81. Welsh F. A., Sims R. E., and Harris V. A. (1990) Mild hypothermia prevents ischemic injury in gerbil hippocampus. *J. Cereb. Blood Flow Metab.* **10,** 557–563.

82. Natale J. A. and D'Alecy L. G. (1989) Protection from cerebral ischemia by brain cooling without reduced lactate accumulation in dogs. *Stroke* **20,** 770–777.

83. Chopp M., Knight R., Tidwell C. D., Helpern J. A., Brown E., and Welch K. M. (1989) The metabolic effects of mild hypothermia on global cerebral ischemia and recirculation in the cat: comparison to normothermia and hyperthermia. *J. Cereb. Blood Flow Metab.* **9,** 141–148.

84. Chen H., Chopp M., Jiang Q., and Garcia J. H. (1992) Neuronal damage, glial response and cerebral metabolism after hypothermic forebrain ischemia in the rat. *Acta Neuropathol.* **84,** 184–189.

85. Ginsberg M. D., Busto R., Castella Y., Valdes I., and Loor J. (1989) The protective effect of moderate intra-ischemic brain hypothermia is associated with improved post-ischemic glucose utilization and blood flow. *J. Cereb. Blood Flow Metab.* **9,** S380.

86. Dietrich W. D., Busto R., Alonso O., Pita-Loor Y., Globus M. Y., and Ginsberg M. D. (1991) Intraischemic brain hypothermia promotes postischemic metabolic recovery and somatosensory circuit activation. *J. Cereb. Blood Flow Metab.* **11,** S846.

87. Rothman S. M. and Olney J. W. (1986) Glutamate and the pathophysiology of hypoxic—ischemic brain damage. *Ann. Neurol.* **19,** 105–111.

88. Choi D. W. and Rothman S. M. (1990) The role of glutamate neurotoxicity in hypoxic-ischemic neuronal death. *Annu. Rev. Neurosci.* **13,** 171–182.

89. Benveniste H. (1991) The excitotoxin hypothesis in relation to cerebral ischemia. *Cerebrovasc. Brain Metab. Rev.* **3,** 213–245.

90. Globus M. Y., Busto R., Dietrich W. D., Martinez E., Valdes I., and Ginsberg M. D. (1988) Effect of ischemia on the in vivo release of striatal dopamine, glutamate, and gamma-aminobutyric acid studied by intracerebral microdialysis. *J. Neurochem.* **51,** 1455–1464.

91. Globus M. Y., Busto R., Dietrich W. D., Martinez E., Valdes I., and Ginsberg M. D. (1989) Direct evidence for acute and massive norepinephrine release in the hippocampus during transient ischemia. *J. Cereb. Blood Flow Metab.* **9,** 892–896.

92. Globus M. Y., Wester P., Busto R., and Dietrich W. D. (1992) Ischemia-induced extracellular release of serotonin plays a role in CA1 neuronal cell death in rats. *Stroke* **23,** 1595–1601.

93. Graf R., Matsumoto K., Risse F., Rosner G., and Heiss W. D. (1992) Effect of mild hypothermia on glutamate accumulation in cat focal ischemia. *Stroke* **23,** 150.

94. Okuda C., Saito A., Miyazaki M., and Kuriyama K. (1986) Alteration of the turnover of dopamine and 5-hydroxytryptamine in rat brain associated with hypothermia. *Pharmacol. Biochem. Behav.* **24,** 79–83.

95. Globus M. Y., Busto R., Dietrich W. D., Martinez E., Valdes I., and Ginsberg M. D. (1988) Intra-ischemic extracellular release of dopamine and glutamate is associated with striatal vulnerability to ischemia. *Neurosci. Lett.* **91,** 36–40.

96. Mitani A. and Kataoka K. (1991) Critical levels of extracellular glutamate mediating gerbil hippocampal delayed neuronal death during hypothermia: brain microdialysis study. *Neuroscience* **42,** 661–670.

97. Baker A. J., Zornow M. H., Grafe M. R., et al. (1991) Hypothermia prevents ischemia-induced increases in hippocampal glycine concentrations in rabbits. *Stroke* **22,** 666–673.

98. Illievich U. M., Zornow M. H., Choi K. T., Scheller M. S., and Strnat M. A. (1994) Effects of hypothermic metabolic suppression on hippocampal glutamate concentrations after transient global cerebral ischemia. *Anesth. Analg.* **78,** 905–911.

99. Illievich U. M., Zornow M. H., Choi K. T., Strnat M. A., and Scheller M. S. (1994) Effects of hypothermia or anesthetics on hippocampal glutamate and glycine concentrations after repeated transient global cerebral ischemia. *Anesthesiology* **80,** 177–186.

100. Li P. A., He Q. P., Miyashita H., Howllet W., Siesjö B. K., and Shuaib A. (1999) Hypothermia ameliorates ischemic brain damage and suppresses the release of extracellular amino acids in both normo- and hyperglycemic subjects. *Exp. Neurol.* **158,** 242–253.

101. Zhao H., Asai S., Kanematsu K., Kunimatsu T., Kohno T., and Ishikawa K. (1997) Real-time monitoring of the effects of normothermia and hypothermia on extracellular glutamate re-uptake in the rat following global brain ischemia. *Neuro-Report* **8,** 2389–2393.

102. Globus M. Y., Busto R., Martinez E., Valdes I., Dietrich W. D., and Ginsberg M. D. (1991) Comparative effect of transient global ischemia on extracellular levels of glutamate, glycine, and gamma-aminobutyric acid in vulnerable and non-vulnerable brain regions in the rat. *J. Neurochem.* **57,** 470–478.

103. Globus M. Y., Busto R., Martinez E., Valdes I., Dietrich W. D., and Ginsberg M. D. (1991) Early moderate postischemic hypothermia attenuates the rise in excitotoxic index in the hippocampus—a possible mechanism for the beneficial effects of postischemic moderate cooling. *J. Cereb. Blood Flow Metab.* **11,** S10.

104. Andine P., Orwar O., Jacobson I., Sandberg M., and Hagberg H. (1991) Changes in extracellular amino acids and spontaneous neuronal activity during ischemia and extended reflow in the CA1 of the rat hippocampus. *J. Neurochem.* **57,** 222–229.

105. Lin B., Globus M. Y., Dietrich W. D., Busto R., Martinez E., and Ginsberg M. D. (1992) Differing neurochemical and morphological sequelae of global ischemia: comparison of single- and multiple-insult paradigms. *J. Neurochem.* **59,** 2213–2223.

106. Busto R., Globus M. Y., Martinez E., Valdes I., and Ginsberg M. D. (1993) Effect of intraischemic hypothermia on ischemia-induced changes in regional levels of inositol 1,4,5-triphosphate (IP$_3$). *Soc. Neurosci. Abstr.* **19,** 1669.

107. Cardell M., Bingren H., Wieloch T., Zivin J., and Saitoh T. (1990) Protein kinase C is translocated to cell membranes during cerebral ischemia. *Neurosci. Lett.* **119,** 228–232.

108. Wieloch T., Cardell M., Bingren H., Zivin J., and Saitoh T. (1991) Changes in the activity of protein kinase C and the differential subcellular redistribution of its isozymes in the rat striatum during and following transient forebrain ischemia. *J. Neurochem.* **56,** 1227–1235.

109. Cardell M., Boris-Moller F., and Wieloch T. (1991) Hypothermia prevents the ischemia-induced translocation and inhibition of protein kinase C in the rat striatum. *J. Neurochem.* **57,** 1814–1817.

110. Harada K., Maekawa T., Tsuruta R., et al. (2002) Hypothermia inhibits translocation of CaM kinase II and PKC-alpha, beta, gamma isoforms and fodrin proteolysis in rat brain synaptosome during ischemia-reperfusion. *J. Neurosci. Res.* **67,** 664–669.

111. Yamashita K., Eguchi Y., Kajiwara K., and Ito H. (1991) Mild hypothermia ameliorates ubiquitin synthesis and prevents delayed neuronal death in the gerbil hippocampus. *Stroke* **22,** 1574–1581.

112. Katsumura H., Kabuto M., Hosotani K., Handa Y., Kobayashi H., and Kubota T. (1995) The influence of total body hyperthermia on brain haemodynamics and blood–brain barrier in dogs. *Acta Neurochir. (Wien)* **135,** 62–69.

113. Dempsey R. J., Combs D. J., Maley M. E., Cowen D. E., Roy M. W., and Donaldson D. L. (1987) Moderate hypothermia reduces postischemic edema development and leukotriene production. *Neurosurgery* **21,** 177–181.

114. Watson B. D. and Ginsberg M. D. (1989) Ischemic injury in the brain. Role of oxygen radical-mediated processes. *Ann. NY Acad. Sci.* **559,** 269–281.

115. Toyoda T., Suzuki S., Kassell N. F., and Lee K. S. (1996) Intraischemic hypothermia attenuates neutrophil infiltration in the rat neocortex after focal ischemia-reperfusion injury. *Neurosurgery* **39,** 1200–1205.

116. Widmann R., Miyazawa T., and Hossmann K. A. (1993) Protective effect of hypothermia on hippocampal injury after 30 minutes of forebrain ischemia in rats is mediated by postischemic recovery of protein synthesis. *J. Neurochem.* **61,** 200–209.

117. Kamme F. and Wieloch T. (1996) The effect of hypothermia on protein synthesis and the expression of immediate early genes following transient cerebral ischemia. *Adv. Neurol.* **71,** 199–206.

118. Kumar K., Wu X., and Evans A. T. (1996) Expression of c-fos and fos-B proteins following transient forebrain ischemia: effect of hypothermia. *Brain Res. Mol. Brain Res.* **42,** 337–343.

119. Zhang Z., Sobel R. A., Cheng D., Steinberg G. K., and Yenari M. A. (2001) Mild hypothermia increases Bcl-2 protein expression following global cerebral ischemia. *Brain Res. Mol. Brain Res.* **95,** 75–85.

120. Boris-Möller F., Kamme F., and Wieloch T. (1998) The effect of hypothermia on the expression of neurotrophin mRNA in the hippocampus following transient cerebral ischemia in the rat. *Brain Res. Mol. Brain Res.* **63,** 163–173.

121. D'Cruz B. J., Fertig K. C., Filiano A. J., Hicks S. D., DeFranco D. B., and Callaway C. W. (2002) Hypothermic reperfusion after cardiac arrest augments brain-derived neurotrophic factor activation. *J. Cereb. Blood Flow Metab.* **22,** 843–851.

3

Mild Hypothermia in Experimental Focal Cerebral Ischemia

Carolina M. Maier, PhD

INTRODUCTION

The majority of acute ischemic strokes occur as a result of thromboembolism of a cerebral artery. The affected brain tissue, the *ischemic core*, is irreversibly damaged rapidly (within 60 min) after the onset of vessel occlusion. A larger area of the brain surrounding the ischemic core, the *ischemic penumbra*, has the potential to recover most of its functions following therapeutic intervention. The initial cell loss is primarily neuronal. However, if the occlusion is extended beyond 1 h, the penumbra begins to be incorporated into the ischemic core, where all cell types are affected. The maturation of damage in the ischemic penumbra may continue for days or weeks. Thus, stroke outcome is determined not only by the volume of the ischemic core, but also by the extent of the secondary brain damage in the penumbra, which is influenced by brain swelling, impaired microcirculation, and inflammation *(1)*.

The mechanisms whereby brain cells die during ischemia are not fully understood. Experimental evidence points to a complex array of parallel hemodynamic, biochemical, and electrophysiological events that combine to produce neuronal damage. In experimental cerebral ischemia, the severity of this damage can be significantly reduced by treatment with mild hypothermia (2–5°C below normal brain temperature).

Although research in this area has been conducted for more than 40 yr, the mechanisms of cerebral protection by mild hypothermia remain unclear and are still a source of controversy. Proposed mechanisms of neuroprotection by mild hypothermia include suppression of neurotransmitter release *(2,3)*, reduced free radical production *(4)*, activity of protein kinases *(5)*, resynthesis of cellular repair proteins *(6)*,

From: *Hypothermia and Cerebral Ischemia: Mechanisms and Clinical Applications*
Edited by: C. M. Maier and G. K. Steinberg © Humana Press Inc., Totowa, NJ

and preservation of the blood–brain barrier (BBB) *(7)*. More recently, there have also been reports that hypothermia may lead to specific inhibition of apoptosis *(8,9)* and the attenuation of the inflammatory response that often follows an ischemic insult *(9–11)*.

The concept of neuroprotection relies on the fact that delayed neuronal injury occurs after ischemia, and each step along the ischemic cascade provides a target for therapeutic intervention. Thus, understanding the cellular and molecular mechanisms that underlie the development of neuronal and vascular injury is critical to optimize treatment. This chapter reviews experimental evidence from studies on focal cerebral ischemia and mild hypothermia, as well as the mechanisms involved in mild hypothermic neuroprotection.

THE ISCHEMIC CASCADE

During cerebral ischemia, energy stores in the brain are depleted within minutes of ischemic onset. Ionic leakage across cell membranes results in edema and persistent membrane depolarization accompanies the release by presynaptic neurons of large amounts of excitatory amino acids (EAAs) such as glutamate and aspartate. The amount of neurotransmitter release correlates with the severity of the ischemic insult and subsequent neuronal injury *(12)*. These neurotransmitters activate postsynaptic receptors, resulting in an increase of intracellular calcium (Ca^{2+}). Intracellular alterations in cytosolic and subcellular calcium dynamics result in the activation of Ca^{2+}-dependent kinases, induction of immediate early genes, and mitochondrial dysfunction *(13)*. Formation of lactic acid causes progressive intracellular acidosis and the release of bound iron—free iron can catabolize free radical formation. Various enzymes are activated (e.g., lipid peroxidases, proteases, phospholipases), increasing intracellular free fatty acids and furthering free radical formation. Caspase, translocase, and endonuclease activity results in DNA fragmentation. What ensues is rapid, necrotic cell death in the ischemic core. In the ischemic penumbra, however, apoptosis (an energy-dependent programmed cell death) likely predominates over necrosis *(14)*. All of these processes result in disintegration of the cell and stimulation of the immune system. Inflammatory and immunological responses also contribute to the pathogenesis of cerebral ischemia. For an in-depth review, see Horst and Korf *(15)*, Sharp et al. *(16)*, and Small et al. *(17)*.

EXPERIMENTAL FOCAL CEREBRAL ISCHEMIA

To be an effective research tool, animal stroke models need to replicate features of human cerebrovascular syndromes. Unlike the clinical situation, experimental animal models allow for high reproducibility and physiological control. Furthermore, they allow for the study of events occurring within the first seconds to minutes of an ischemic insult, which are critical to our understanding of the pathophysiology of stroke *(18)*. In focal cerebral ischemia, the most commonly used animal model involves middle cerebral artery occlusion (MCAO) either by directly ligating or clipping the vessel, or by introducing an intraluminal suture via the carotid artery. This allows either permanent or transient occlusions (also referred to as ischemia/reperfusion [I/R]). Other focal cerebral ischemia models include photochemically induced focal cerebral thrombosis *(19)* and blood clot embolization *(20,21)*. Detailed reviews of these models can be found in McAuley *(22)* and Ginsberg and Busto *(18)*.

Despite efforts at standardization, a major problem with early cerebral ischemia experiments was the extent of variability in neuronal damage depending on the animal model used, the chosen animal species (normotensive vs spontaneously hypertensive animals), duration of vessel occlusion, and brain area examined. Furthermore, in such early experiments, rectal temperature was considered sufficient for monitoring, and brain temperature was rarely measured. In the 1980s, Busto and colleagues demonstrated variability in cerebral versus scalp temperatures in animals undergoing carotid artery occlusion with hypotension. They subsequently showed that small differences in intraischemic brain temperature (1–2°C) critically determined the extent of ischemic neuronal injury *(23)*. That study led to a variety of experimental paradigms designed to test the optimal depth, duration, and long-term effects of mild hypothermic treatment in stroke. Representative studies on focal cerebral ischemia can be seen in **Table 1**.

When studying the effects of temperature modulations, one must keep in mind that brain temperature is not uniform. Various animal studies have shown that there is a temperature gradient between deep and superficial brain tissues *(24–26)*. The first reason for this gradient is that superficial brain tissues with their supplying arterial vessels lose heat to their surroundings. Heat loss in the brain can occur through simple evaporation— such as from mucous membranes in the nasal and oral cavities *(27)*. This means that even deep tissues can lose heat to their surroundings.

Table 1
Representative Studies on Focal Cerebral Ischemia

Reference	Species	Ischemia model	Duration	Hypothermia groups (°C)	Measures	Effects of hypothermia
Lo and Steinberg, 1992	New Zealand White rabbits	Anterior and MCAo, ICAo	Permanent	37, 33, 30; 4 h intraischemia	Somatosensory evoked potentials, regional blood flow, MRI at 4 h	Recovery of evoked potentials, reduced blood flow, reduced T1 and T2 relaxation times in MRI
Kader et al., 1992	Wistar rats	MCAo	Permanent	30, 33, 34.5, 36.5, 1 h intraischemia, and 33, 1 h postischemia	Infarct volume 24 h postischemia	Reduced infarct volume in all hypothermia groups
Ridenour et al., 1992	SH Rats	MCAo	Permanent or 1 h temporary	33 and 37; 2 h intraischemia, 1 h intraischemia, or 1 h postischemia	Infarct volume 96 h postischemia and neurologic function 24 h and 96 h postischemia	No change in infarct for permanent MCAo, reduced infarct for temporary MCAo, no clear effect on function
Baker et al., 1995	Wistar rats	MCAo	Permanent	33 and 37 intraischemia	Cortical glutamate concentration (in vivo microdialysis), and infarct volume	Reduced glutamate release and infarct volume

Winfree et al., 1996	Wistar rats	MCAo	Permanent	33 and 37 intraischemia	Penumbral glutamate concentration (in vivo microdialysis), CBF, and infarct volume 2 h postischemia	Reduced glutamate release, no change in CBF, reduced infarct volume
Frazzini et al., 1994	Wistar rats	MCAo	Permanent	33 and 37, intraischemia, with or without MK-801 before or after ischemia	Infarct volume 24 h postischemia	Both hypothermia and MK-801 reduced infarct size; no further reduction when combined
Maier et al., 2002	SD rats	MCAo	1 h or 2 h (or 90 min in some rats) with reperfusion	33 and 37, intraischemia	Superoxide anion production, SOD expression and activity, 0 h to 2 mo postischemia	Reduced superoxide production in penumbra, no change in SOD expression, slight reduction in SOD activity
Wang et al., 2002	SD rats	MCAo	2 h, with reperfusion	33 and 37, intraischemia	Infarct size, ICAM-1 expression, neutrophil and monocyte infiltration, microglial activation at 1 d, 3 d, and 7 d postischemia	Reduced infarct size, ICAM-1, neutrophils and monocytes, and microglial activation
Maier et al., 2001	SD rats	MCAo	90 min or 2 h, with reperfusion	33 and 37, intraischemia or delayed up to 1 h postreperfusion	Infarct size at 3 d, 7 d, 2 mo, neurologic function at 1 d, 2 d, and at final end point	Reduced infarct size, improved neurologic function, sustained over 2 mo

43

(continued)

Table 1 (*continued*)

Reference	Species	Ischemia model	Duration	Hypothermia groups (°C)	Measures	Effects of hypothermia
Maier et al., 1998	SD rats	MCAo	2 h, with reperfusion	30, 33, and 37, during first 30 min, 1 h, or 2 h of ischemia	Infarct size, neurologic function, apoptosis (TUNEL stain, morphology, DNA fragmentation), inflammation (MPO stain) 1 d and 3 d postreperfusion	Reduced infarct size, improved neurologic function, reduced apoptosis and inflammation with 1 h or 2 h hypothermia
Markarian et al., 1996	SD rats	MCAo and bilateral carotid occlusion	3 h, with reperfusion	32–33 and 36–37, for 1–4 h intra- and postischemia or delayed 15, 30, or 45 min after ischemia onset	Infarct volume	Reduced infarct volume (larger reductions with longer hypothermia), less effective when delayed 45 min
Kader et al., 1994	Wistar rats	MCAo and bilateral carotid occlusion	Permanent, lasting 0, 10, 20, or 60 min followed by death	33 and 36.5, intraischemia	Nitrite levels, cGMP levels, NOS activity during ischemia	Reduced nitrite and cGMP levels, reduced NOS activity

Kumura et al., 1996	SD rats	MCAo	2 h, with reperfusion	32, 34, 37, and 39, intraischemia	Jugular nitric oxide during reperfusion	Reduced jugular nitric oxide levels
Goto, 1993	SD rats	MCAo and bilateral carotid occlusion	3 h, with reperfusion	~28, 33, and 36, intraischemia	Infarct volume 3 d postischemia	Reduced infarct volume (larger reduction at lower temperature)
Kozlowski et al., 1997	SH rats	Right CCAo and MCAo	CCAo permanent and MCAo either permanent or transient (3 h)	32 and 37.5, intraischemia	Infarct volume, pH, NAA, high-energy phosphates during ischemia and reperfusion	No effect in permanent occlusion; reduced infarct, improved recovery in metabolite levels during reperfusion
Chen et al., 1992	Wistar rats	MCAo	2 h, with reperfusion	30 and 37, intraischemia	Neuronal damage, astrocyte damage, and inflammation 4 d postischemia	Reduced neuronal damage, astrocytic reaction, and inflammatory response
Kil et al., 1996	SD rats	Bilateral CCAo with hypotension	15 min, with 60 min reperfusion	30, 36, and 39, intraischemia	Hydroxyl radical production, CBF	Reduced hydroxyl radical production, no change in CBF
Onesti et al., 1991	SH rats	MCAo	Permanent	24 and 36, intraischemia and 1 h postischemia	Infarct volume 24 h postischemia	Reduced infarct size
Morikawa et al., 1992	SD rats	MCAo	Permanent, permanent with hypotension, 2 h transient	30, 36, and 39, intraischemic	Infarct area and CBF 3 d postischemia	No change in infarct area in permanent MCAo groups, reduced infarct in transient group

(continued)

Table 1 (*continued*)

Reference	Species	Ischemia model	Duration	Hypothermia groups (°C)	Measures	Effects of hypothermia
Lo et al., 1993	New Zealand White rabbits	Anterior and MCAo, ICAo	Permanent	33 and 37.5, intraischemia	Extracellular amino acid levels over 4 h, infarct volume at 4 h postischemia	Reduced glutamate, increased alanine, no other amino acid changes, no change in infarct volume
Chen et al., 1993	Wistar rats	MCAo	90 min transient	30, 37, and 40, intraischemia and 1 h postischemia	Cortical electrical activity, infarct volume 7 d postischemia	Reduced cerebral depolarization during ischemia, reduced infarct volume
Nakashima and Todd, 1996	SD rats	Global ischemia (cardiac arrest)	Permanent	25, 31, 34, and 38, intraischemia	Cortical electrical activity, EAA and GABA release during ischemia	Time to depolarization increased, decreased chemical levels, larger effect of lower body temperatures
Hildebrandt-Eriksen et al., 2002	Wistar rats	CCAo and distal MCAo	30 min	34 and 37, intraischemia	Infarct volume at 14 d postischemia, development of infarct tracked with MRI daily	Reduced infarct volume
Kollmar et al., 2002	SD rats	MCAo	2 h, with 5 h reperfusion	33 only during reperfusion; managed arterial CO_2 tension at 40 mmHg (α-stat) OR corrected it for hypothermia (pH-stat)	CBF, infarct volume, edema at 5 h reperfusion	pH-stat reduced infarct volume and edema, increased CBF

46

Reference	Species	Model	Ischemia	Temperature (°C)	Outcome measures	Results
Yunoki et al., 2002	SD rats	Bilateral CCAo and MCAo	1 h, with reperfusion	25.5, 28.5, and 31.5 for 20 min 24 h preischemia, OR 33 and 34.5 for 20, 60, 120, or 180 min 24 h preischemia, OR 28.5 and 31.5 head-only (hypothermic preconditioning)	Infarct volume 24 h postischemia	Tolerance to ischemia (reduced infarct volume) greater with cooler, longer hypothermia, and restricted hypothermia effective as global hypothermia
Nishio et al., 2002	Cats	MCAo	1 h, with reperfusion	30.5 and 36.5, intraischemia plus 3 h, with slow or rapid rewarming	Somatosensory evoked potentials (SEPs), edema at 5 h reperfusion	Edema reduced in hypothermia with slow rewarming, recovery of SEPs enhanced with slow rewarming
Kollmar et al., 2002	Wistar rats	MCAo	2 h, with reperfusion	33 and 37, started 1 h after reperfusion	MRI, neurological function, edema, infarct volume, 1–5 d postischemia	Increased survival, improved neurological function, reduced edema, reduced infarct volume
Wainwright et al., 2002	SD rats	MCAo	70 min or 120 min, with or without hemoglobin O_2 binding affinity restored by RSR13	30, 34, and 37	Infarct volume, neurological function 7 d postischemia	Reduced infarct volume and improved neurological function; RSR13 had no effect

(continued)

Table 1 *(continued)*

Reference	Species	Ischemia model	Duration	Hypothermia groups (°C)	Measures	Effects of hypothermia
Yenari et al., 2002	SD rats	MCAo	2 h, with reperfusion	33–34 and 37, intraischemia	Infarct size, Bcl-2 and Bax expression, mitochondrial cytochrome c release, caspase activation 2–72 h postischemia	Reduced infarct size, reduced cytochrome c release, no effect on other proteins or caspase activation

CBF, Cerebral blood flow; CCAo, common carotid artery occlusion; cGMP, cyclic guanine monophosphate; ICAM-1, intercellular adhesion molecule-1; ICAo, internal carotid artery occlusion; MCAo, middle cerebral artery occlusion; NAA, *N*-acetyl-aspartate; NOS, nitric oxide synthase; SD, Sprague–Dawley; SH, spontaneously hypertensive; SOD, superoxide dismutase; TUNEL, transferase dUTP nick-end labeling.

Brain temperature also depends on regional cerebral blood flow (rCBF). Following vascular occlusion, deep brain tissues may suffer a transient temperature rise reflecting the failure of arterial blood to remove metabolic heat *(28)*. As superficial tissues cool, the temperature in deep tissues also decreases. Thus, by retarding or interrupting blood flow, ischemia upsets temperature regulation.

Mild hypothermia has been shown to reduce neurological deficits if started before, during, or after cerebral ischemia, but few studies have examined functional outcome in detail after experimental cerebral ischemia with hypothermia *(29–33)*.

To understand the effects of mild hypothermia on neurological outcome following a focal insult and to determine the optimal depth of hypothermic treatment, we studied rats that underwent 2 h of MCAO followed by 24–72 h of reperfusion *(9)*. Mild (33°C) hypothermia did not produce the systemic complications, including decreased respiratory rate and cardiac arrhythmias, that were observed in animals treated with moderate (30°C) hypothermia. In addition, animals in the 33°C group recovered from anesthesia at a significantly faster rate than those treated with 30°C. This suggested that mild hypothermia might be a safer, more manageable alternative to moderate hypothermia.

The optimal duration of intraischemic hypothermia was also addressed in that study. Both 1 and 2 h of intraischemic hypothermia, started at the onset of ischemia, were sufficient to reduce the behavioral and histopathological deficits associated with transient focal cerebral ischemia. Thirty minutes of mild hypothermia, however, was not effective in either outcome measure. Other reports show conflicting results. Kader et al. *(34)* found that 33°C or 34.5°C for 1 h, induced at onset of ischemia, reduced infarction due to permanent MCAO with a 24-h endpoint. Another study, however, found that 33°C for 1 h duration reduced infarct size at 4 d after transient but not permanent focal ischemia. Karibe et al. *(35)* found a significant reduction in infarction if mild intraischemic hypothermia was introduced within 30 min of transient (2 h) MCAO, but the protection was lost if hypothermic induction was delayed by more than 60 min. Thus, while it may not be necessary to maintain intraischemic hypothermia for more than 1 h if started within 30 min of focal ischemic onset, longer time periods of hypothermia are likely needed to achieve neuroprotection following permanent vessel occlusion or if initiated in a delayed fashion after ischemic onset.

A critical factor in developing a therapeutic strategy against stroke is the time window available. In focal cerebral ischemia, delaying the

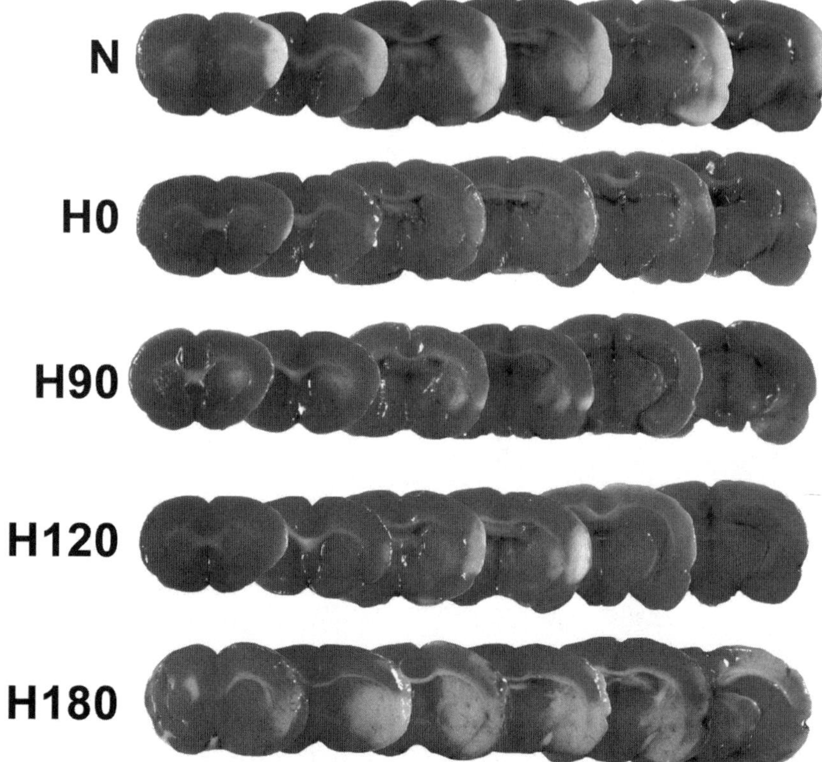

Fig. 1. Coronal sections from representative normothermic (N) animals and animals treated with 2 h of hypothermia (33°C) started at ischemia onset (H0) or with delays of 90 (H90), 120 (H120), or 180 (H180) min and allowed to survive for 3 d following 2-h MCAO. The coronal sections were incubated in 2% triphenyltetrazolium chloride (TTC) at 37°C for 15 min. *Dark areas* indicate viable tissue while *pale areas* indicate infarcted tissue.

onset of mild hypothermia (1- to 3-h duration) up to 1.5 h (but not beyond) has shown benefits *(35–38)*. Initiating treatment 2 h after ischemia (2-h MCAO) onset has also shown benefits *(39)*, but only if hypothermia (32°C) is maintained for a 3-h period followed by an additional 2-h period at 35°C.

We recently carried out a study *(40)* to determine the effects of delaying induction of mild hypothermia after transient focal cerebral ischemia and to ascertain whether the neuroprotective effects of mild hypothermia induced during the ischemic period are sustained over

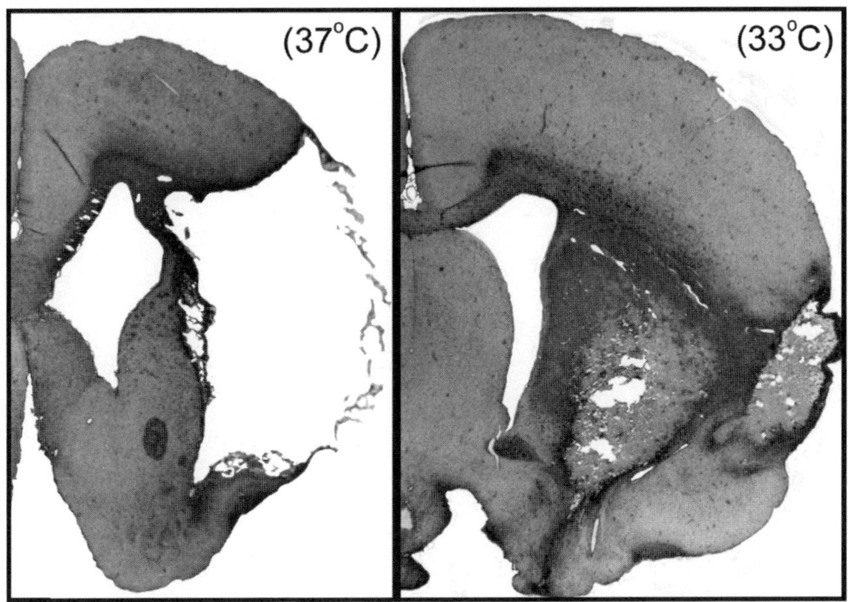

Fig. 2. Representative coronal sections of a normothermic and a hypothermic animal 2 mo after 2-h MCAO. Although there is no tissue left in the infarcted area of the normothermic animal, the periinfarct zone still shows reactive astrocytes expressing glial fibrillary acidic protein (GFAP) and manganese-superoxide dismutase (SOD2) which can be seen as a *dark rim* around the infarcted area. The hypothermia-treated animal shows a significantly smaller infarct.

time. We found that mild hypothermia conferred significant degrees of neuroprotection in terms of survival, behavioral deficits, and histopathological changes, even when its induction was delayed by 120 min after MCAO onset (**Fig. 1**). Furthermore, the neuroprotection of mild hypothermia (2-h duration) that was induced during the ischemia period was sustained over 2 mo (**Fig. 2**). Our results differed from those of Yanamoto et al. *(38)*, who had shown that, in response to mild hypothermic conditions maintained during ischemia (2 h) and postischemia (3 h), the reduction in infarct volume observed at 2 d post-MCAO was lost at 30 d postocclusion. However, maintaining hypothermia for an additional 21 h postsurgery had long-lasting benefits. The same group had previously shown a significant reduction in infarct volume in cases where mild hypothermia was induced immediately on reperfusion and maintained for 21 h, whereas an immediate but brief (1-h) period of hypothermia was ineffective *(37)*.

The time window for the therapeutic effectiveness of hypothermia (2 h after ischemia onset) may appear to be relatively narrow, offering potential benefit in a controlled intraoperative surgical setting *(41)*, but being less applicable for treating patients suffering from spontaneous stroke. However, combination therapy using mild hypothermia and pharmacological intervention may be efficacious (for details *see* Chapter 6).

The main role of mild hypothermia against stroke may, perhaps, be to extend the therapeutic window of other treatment modalities. On the other hand, hypothermia is by far the most potent neuroprotectant available against experimental cerebral ischemia, and new technological advances are now facilitating its implementation in the clinical setting. Understanding the mechanisms by which mild hypothermia exerts its neuroprotective effects will allow us to optimize its use as a therapeutic strategy.

MECHANISMS UNDERLYING HYPOTHERMIC NEUROPROTECTION

Cerebral Metabolism and Blood Flow

When mild hypothermia was first shown to be beneficial, the assumption was that a substantial portion of its neuroprotective effect stemmed from a reduction in cerebral metabolism. However, studies on cerebral metabolic rate (CMR) made it clear that the degree of neuropathological injury following ischemia with mild hypothermic treatment did not correlate with the magnitude of metabolic depression observed *(42)*. A reduction in temperature from 37°C to 34°C produces a 15–20% reduction in cerebral metabolism (approx 5–7% per °C), which is far less than the 50% decrease seen with electroencephalogram (EEG) silence. Furthermore, reductions in metabolism produced by anesthetics vs hypothermia are not equally neuroprotective *(43)*. Thus, hypothermic neuroprotection cannot be explained by alterations in metabolic rate alone.

Data on the hemodynamic consequences of hypothermia show conflicting results depending on the cooling method used (systemic vs local), the degree of hypothermia produced, and the duration of hypothermic treatment *(35,44–47)*. In a permanent focal ischemia model, hypothermia (30°C) has been shown to reduce cortical CBF relative to 37°C or 33°C *(48)*. In that study, alterations in regional CBF were not observed in other brain regions. Because blood pressure is a critical determinant of infarct size—raising blood pressure improves collateral blood flow and reduces stroke size—it is counterintuitive to think that a reduction in blood flow might be beneficial. However, other studies on transient MCAO *(35,49)* suggest that mild hypothermia may inhibit postischemic hyperperfusion and delayed or sustained hypoperfusion in ischemic perifocal regions. Yanamoto et al. *(50)* showed that prolonged (24-h duration) mild hypothermic treatment following permanent MCAO decreased infarct volume and spontaneously increased regional CBF.

The effect of hypothermia on CBF may also be dependent on acid–base management during hypothermic treatment *(51,52)*. Following 2 h of normothermic MCAO and 5 h of hypothermic (33°C) reperfusion, Kollmar et al. *(52)* showed that pH-stat management significantly decreased cerebral infarct volume and edema, probably by increasing CBF.

Taking these data into account, it is difficult to believe that the neuroprotective effects of hypothermia are due mainly to alterations in metabolic rate or CBF. On the other hand, it seems reasonable to think that hypothermia reduces membrane functions that are critical for the development of ischemic neuronal damage.

Hypothermia and EAAs

Several groups have shown that mild hypothermia attenuates ischemia-induced EAA release. Following global ischemia, glutamate levels increase within 10–20 min of ischemia onset, then decrease by 30–50 min *(2,53–56)*. Following focal cerebral ischemia, glutamate levels typically peak within 60 min of ischemia onset, then return to baseline levels *(57,58)* or decrease substantially *(59)* by 90–120 min. A few groups have shown that mild hypothermia is still effective even when applied after glutamate peaks (delayed by 60–120 min) *(36,39,40, 60,61)*. The decrease in glutamate release under ischemic conditions with hypothermic treatment is an important mechanism for neuronal protection. However, this reduction in glutamate is not the only mechanism of protection, as it cannot explain the decrease in neuronal damage when hypothermia is applied up to 3 h postinsult.

Neurotransmitters such as glutamate interact with a variety of receptors that are coupled to second messenger systems. The effects of mild hypothermia on ischemia-induced changes in intracellular messenger systems and mediators have also been studied and are described in Chapter 2.

BBB and Cerebral Edema

Formation of cerebral edema caused by vascular leakage accounts for much of the morbidity and mortality associated with stroke. Brain edema can be either intracellular (cytotoxic edema) or interstitial (vasogenic edema). The initial hypoxic insult suffered by cells during an ischemic event results primarily in cytotoxic edema, while vasogenic edema is seen on reperfusion. Disruption of the BBB contributes to brain injury by allowing the passage of potentially harmful blood-borne substances into the brain parenchyma. Hypothermia has been shown to reduce BBB breakdown, thus limiting the passage of such substances across the endothelial barrier and subsequent vasogenic edema *(62,63)*. A recent study by Kollmar et al. *(64)* showed that even delayed postischemic hypothermia (33°C initiated 3 h post-MCAO, 5-h duration) could reduce the extent of cerebral edema as evaluated by serial magnetic resonance imaging (MRI) over a 5-d period. Amelioration of cytotoxic edema by mild hypothermia is also very likely when the hypothermic reduction of glutamate surge, calcium mobilization, and ATP expenditure are taken into consideration *(61,65)*. There is also evidence suggesting that the opening and closing of water and ion channels are carefully regulated by temperature *(66)*.

Free Radicals and Inflammation

Recent evidence suggests that oxygen free radicals may play a significant role in the development of microvascular damage and subsequent breakdown of the BBB. There is reason to believe that mild hypothermia may exert its protective effects by directly altering processes such as the generation of reactive oxygen species (ROS). Ischemic injury may evolve over a period of days *(67)*, with secondary injury resulting from ROS generated from resident brain cells and leukocytes *(40,68)*. There are many sources of ROS, including the mitochondrial electron transport chain and activated leukocytes *(69)*. ROS, which can be generated soon after hypoxia/ischemia *(70)* as well as in later stages during postischemic reperfusion *(71)*, can attack the major cellular components and alter membrane functions. Several reports have documented a decrease in free radical generation following reperfusion with lower brain temperature *(4,72–75)* and a reduction in infiltrating brain neutrophils *(9,10)*. Consistent with this is the observation by some clinicians that hypothermia may be related to an increase in incidence of infections, especially with cooling periods longer than 24 h *(75)*.

To examine the effects of mild hypothermia on the cellular and molecular events associated with the production of ROS implicated in ischemia-induced neuronal damage, we have used a 2-h MCAO model and survival times up to 2 mo postinsult *(4)*. By means of free radical fluorescence, we have shown that mild intraischemic hypothermia significantly reduces the generation of superoxide (O_2^-), a free radical that is directly toxic to neurons *(76)*, in peri-infarct areas. We have also shown that O_2^- is produced primarily in neurons and endothelial cells, although some O_2^- production is occasionally observed in oligodendrocytes with this model.

A second source of ROS in later stages of postischemic reperfusion is activated leukocytes *(69)*. We have previously shown that mild hypothermia may act by reducing the number of infiltrating leukocytes, thus attenuating the generation of ROS that occurs several days following transient MCAO *(9)*. A transient MCAO study by Toyoda et al. *(10)* using myeloperoxidase (MPO) activity to assess leukocyte levels also showed that intraischemic hypothermia attenuated leukocyte accumulation and produced a 59% reduction in infarct volume compared to normothermia. Similar results have also been obtained in a model of thrombin-induced edema formation *(62)*.

Additional evidence linking hypothermia and highly reactive free radicals comes from studies on endogenous antioxidants in brain tissue. Karibe et al. *(77)* showed that following 3 h of MCAO, intraischemic mild hypothermia suppresses the reduction of cortical tissue concentrations of the endogenous antioxidants ascorbate and glutathione detected 3 h into reperfusion. Based on the observation that expression of free radical scavengers such as superoxide dismutase (SOD, the enzymatic scavenger of O_2^-) increases following an ischemic insult *(78,79)*, Fukuhara et al. *(80)* examined the induction of the cytosolic isoform of SOD (Cu/Zn-SOD or SOD1) in rats 6 h after cerebral contusion under hypothermia. Results showed an increase in SOD1 messenger RNA in the periphery of the contusion and decreased brain edema in hypothermic animals.

We have also studied the expression and activity of SOD under normothermic and hypothermic conditions in a transient MCAO model *(4)* and found that SOD activity was nearly identical in the noninfarcted tissue of normothermic and hypothermic animals. There were no significant differences in enzyme activity between temperature groups in the ischemic cortex; however, SOD activity was slightly reduced in the ischemic striatum (infarct core) of hypothermia-treated animals at 2 h with a similar trend at 24 h postinsult. In that study, there was a robust increase in SOD activity at 24 h relative to the 2-h time point in all animals, lending further support to the notion that oxidative processes play a very significant role in infarct development. Neutrophils are a significant source of ROS. These cells begin to infiltrate the infarcted tissue 6–24 h after ischemia, followed by a massive invasion of monocytes at 2–3 d postinsult (68). A decrease in neutrophil infiltration in hypothermia-treated animals (40) may induce a less robust antioxidant response in these animals, and could therefore explain the small decrease in striatal SOD activity observed in hypothermic animals compared with normothermic controls. Thus, although mild intraischemic hypothermia does not appear to alter SOD expression, it does reduce the levels of $O_2{}^-$ produced during the first hour of reperfusion following transient focal cerebral ischemia.

Aside from ROS, inflammatory cells also generate potentially damaging nitric oxide (NO) and cytokines. Cytokines activate microglia and stimulate expression of adhesion molecules leading to leukocyte infiltration. NO and $O_2{}^-$ are highly reactive chemical species that can also combine to form peroxynitrite, a particularly damaging reactive species. Using a 2-h MCAO model, Han et al. (11) showed that mild hypothermia (2-h duration), applied immediately or 2 h after MCAO onset, could inhibit the inflammatory response by affecting microglial-associated inducible nitric oxide synthase (iNOS) and subsequent generation of nitric oxide (NO) and peroxynitrite. This neuroprotective mechanism by mild hypothermia is particularly important, as microglial activation is a delayed and long-lasting phenomenon after ischemia that is believed to contribute to cerebral ischemic damage (81). Work by the same group also showed that postischemic hypothermia (2-h delay) is a more potent inhibitor of neuronal NOS (nNOS) and iNOS expression compared to intraischemic hypothermia, in spite of equivalent protection in an MCAO model (82).

Genetic Models

The development of genetically manipulated laboratory mice deficient in or overexpressing enzymes/proteins in the free radical pathways has allowed substantial progress to be made in stroke research. An example is knockout (KO) mice with targeted disruption of the inducible SOD (Mn-SOD or SOD2). The development of these animals has provided a model for studying the effects of free radicals by perturbing the enzymatic machinery responsible for their metabolism. Using SOD2–KO mice, which are more susceptible to ischemic damage than their wild-type counterparts, we have been able to test simultaneously the efficacy of mild hypothermia and determine if SOD2 expression is critical for the neuroprotection afforded by small temperature reductions. We have found that SOD2–KO mice treated with mild intra-ischemic hypothermia (33°C) have not only a significant reduction in infarct size at 3 d post-MCAO, but also a reduction in the rate of hemorrhagic transformations compared to the normothermic animals *(83)*.

Gene Expression

Cerebral ischemia leads to induction of a number of different genes. Among them are immediate early genes, many of which code for transcription factors *(84)*. Hypothermia has been shown to affect transcriptional events with considerable regional and temporal variability (for a complete review see Kamme and Wieloch *[85]*). Following 1 h of focal cerebral ischemia, mild hypothermia has also been shown to alter the expression of antiapoptotic proteins (e.g., Bcl-2) and proapoptotic proteins (e.g., Bax) *(86)*. On the other hand, using a 2-h MCAO model, Yenari et al. *(87)* showed that mild intraischemic hypothermia did not alter Bcl-2 and Bax expression, but it significantly decreased the amount of cytochrome *c* release 5 h after the onset of ischemia. Mitochondrial release of cytochrome *c* has recently been shown to be a key trigger in caspase activation and apoptosis via the intrinsic pathway. The study by Yenari et al. provided the first evidence that intraischemic mild hypothermia could attenuate the release of cytochrome *c* in the brain, while at the same time not affecting the biochemical aspects of the intrinsic apoptotic pathway. Their results suggest that necrotic processes following cerebral ischemia may have been interrupted to prevent cytochrome *c* release, and that the ameliorative effect of mild hypothermia may be a result of maintaining mitochondrial integrity. A mild hypothermia study using an in vitro model of serum deprivation, which results primarily in apoptotic cell death, has also confirmed these findings *(88)*.

CONCLUSIONS

A large effort examining the potential efficacy of mild hypothermia to protect neurons from ischemic injury has shown promise in experimental stroke models and is now being translated into clinical trials. To develop the use of mild hypothermia as an efficacious and safe therapy against cerebral ischemic damage, it is vital to elucidate the cellular and molecular mechanisms that control neuronal and vascular injury and the effects that altering temperature may have on them. These mechanisms include the excitotoxic cascade, the pathways of free radical injury, the independent mechanisms of programmed cell death, signal transduction pathways, intracellular pH, induction of immediate early genes, and mitochondrial function, to name a few. The scope and range of potential intervention by mild hypothermia in stroke is vast, yet dependent on our understanding of the pathophysiology of cerebral ischemia.

ACKNOWLEDGMENTS

This work was supported by grants from the National Institutes of Health (NIH-NINDS) and American Heart Association. The author thanks Dr. David Schaal for editorial assistance and Beth Hoyte for preparation of the figures.

REFERENCES

1. Stanimirovic D. and Satoh K. (2000) Inflammatory mediators of cerebral endothelium: a role in ischemic brain inflammation. *Brain Pathol.* **10,** 113–126.
2. Busto R., Globus M. Y., Dietrich W. D., Martinez E., Valdes I., and Ginsberg M. D. (1989) Effect of mild hypothermia on ischemia-induced release of neurotransmitters and free fatty acids in rat brain. *Stroke* **20,** 904–910.
3. Patel P. M., Drummond J. C., Cole D. J., and Yaksh T. L. (1994) Differential temperature sensitivity of ischemia-induced glutamate release and eicosanoid production in rats. *Brain Res.* **650,** 205–211.
4. Maier C. M., Sun G. H., Cheng D., Yenari M. A., Chan P. H., and Steinberg G. K. (2002) Effects of mild hypothermia on superoxide anion production, superoxide dismutase expression, and activity following transient focal cerebral ischemia. *Neurobiol. Dis.* **11,** 28–42.
5. Cardell M., Boris-Moller F., and Wieloch T. (1991) Hypothermia prevents the ischemia-induced translocation and inhibition of protein kinase C in the rat striatum. *J. Neurochem.* **57,** 1814–1817.
6. Yamashita K., Eguchi Y., Kajiwara K., and Ito H. (1991) Mild hypothermia ameliorates ubiquitin synthesis and prevents delayed neuronal death in the gerbil hippocampus. *Stroke* **22,** 1574–1581.
7. Dietrich W. D., Busto R., Halley M., and Valdes I. (1990) The importance of brain temperature in alterations of the blood-brain barrier following cerebral ischemia. *J. Neuropathol. Exp. Neurol.* **49,** 486–497.
8. Edwards A. D., Yue X., Squier M. V., et al. (1995) Specific inhibition of apoptosis after cerebral hypoxia-ischaemia by moderate post-insult hypothermia. *Biochem. Biophys. Res. Commun.* **217,** 1193–1199.
9. Maier C. M., Ahern K., Cheng M. L., Lee J. E., Yenari M. A., and Steinberg G. K. (1998) Optimal depth and duration of mild hypothermia in a focal model of transient

cerebral ischemia: effects on neurologic outcome, infarct size, apoptosis, and inflammation. *Stroke* **29,** 2171–2180.

10. Toyoda T., Suzuki S., Kassell N. F., and Lee K. S. (1996) Intraischemic hypothermia attenuates neutrophil infiltration in the rat neocortex after focal ischemia–reperfusion injury. *Neurosurgery* **39,** 1200–1205.

11. Han H. S., Qiao Y., Karabiyikoglu M., Giffard R. G., and Yenari M. A. (2002) Influence of mild hypothermia on inducible nitric oxide synthase expression and reactive nitrogen production in experimental stroke and inflammation. *J. Neurosci.* **22,** 3921–3928.

12. Choi D. W. (1988) Glutamate neurotoxicity and diseases of the nervous system. *Neuron* **1,** 623–634.

13. Luiten P. G. M., Stuiver B., de Jong G. I., Nyakas C., and De Keyser J. H. A. (1997) Calcium homeostasis, nimodipine, and stroke. In *Clinical Pharmacology of Cerebral Ischemia* (Ter Horst G. J. and Korf J., eds.), Humana Press, Totowa, NJ, pp. 67–99.

14. Martin L. J., Al-Abdulla N. A., Brambrink A. M., Kirsch J. R., Sieber F. E., and Portera-Cailliau C. (1998) Neurodegeneration in excitotoxicity, global cerebral ischemia, and target deprivation: a perspective on the contributions of apoptosis and necrosis. *Brain Res. Bull.* **46,** 281–309.

15. Horst G. J. T. and Korf J. (1997) *Clinical Pharmacology of Cerebral Ischemia.* Humana Press, Totowa, NJ.

16. Sharp F. R., Lu A., Tang Y., and Millhorn D. E. (2000) Multiple molecular penumbras after focal cerebral ischemia. *J. Cereb. Blood Flow Metab.* **20,** 1011–1032.

17. Small D. L., Morley P., and Buchan A. M. (1999) Biology of ischemic cerebral cell death. *Prog. Cardiovasc. Dis.* **42,** 185–207.

18. Ginsberg M. D. and Busto R. (1989) Rodent models of cerebral ischemia. *Stroke* **20,** 1627–1642.

19. Nagai N., Zhao B. Q., Suzuki Y., Ihara H., Urano T., and Umemura K. (2002) Tissue-type plasminogen activator has paradoxical roles in focal cerebral ischemic injury by thrombotic middle cerebral artery occlusion with mild or severe photo-chemical damage in mice. *J. Cereb. Blood Flow Metab.* **22,** 648–651.

20. Meden P., Overgaard K., Pedersen H., and Boysen G. (1994) The influence of body temperature on infarct volume and thrombolytic therapy in a rat embolic stroke model. *Brain Res.* **647,** 131–138.

21. Meden P., Overgaard K., Pedersen H., and Boysen G. (1994) Effect of hypothermia and delayed thrombolysis in a rat embolic stroke model. *Acta Neurol. Scand.* **90,** 91–98.

22. McAuley M. A. (1995) Rodent models of focal ischemia. *Cerebrovasc. Brain Metab. Rev.* **7,** 153–180.

23. Busto R., Dietrich W. D., Globus M. Y., Valdes I., Scheinberg P., and Ginsberg M. D. (1987) Small differences in intraischemic brain temperature critically determine the extent of ischemic neuronal injury. *J. Cereb. Blood Flow Metab.* **7,** 729–738.

24. Delgado J. M. and Hanai T. (1966) Intracerebral temperatures in free-moving cats. *Am. J. Physiol.* **211,** 755–769.

25. Ward T. R., Svensgaard D. J., Spiegel R. J., Puckett E. T., Long M. D., and Kinn J. B. (1986) Brain temperature measurements in rats: a comparison of microwave and ambient temperature exposures. *Bioelectromagnetics* **7,** 243–258.

26. Williams W. M., Lu S. T., Del Cerro M., and Michaelson S. M. (1984) Effect of 2450 MHz microwave energy on the blood–brain barrier to hydrophilic molecules.

D. Brain temperature and blood–brain barrier permeability to hydrophilic tracers. *Brain Res.* **319,** 191–212.

27. Minamisawa H., Mellergard P., Smith M. L., et al. (1990) Preservation of brain temperature during ischemia in rats. *Stroke* **21,** 758–764.

28. Hayward J. N. and Baker M. A. (1969) A comparative study of the role of the cerebral arterial blood in the regulation of brain temperature in five mammals. *Brain Res.* **16,** 417–440.

29. Corbett D., Nurse S., and Colbourne F. (1997) Hypothermic neuroprotection. A global ischemia study using 18- to 20-month-old gerbils. *Stroke* **28,** 2238–2242.

30. Colbourne F. and Corbett D. (1995) Delayed postischemic hypothermia: a six month survival study using behavioral and histological assessments of neuroprotection. *J. Neurosci.* **15,** 7250–7260.

31. Nurse S. and Corbett D. (1994) Direct measurement of brain temperature during and after intraischemic hypothermia: correlation with behavioral, physiological, and histological endpoints. *J. Neurosci.* **14,** 7726–7734.

32. Green E. J., Dietrich W. D., van Dijk F., et al. (1992) Protective effects of brain hypothermia on behavior and histopathology following global cerebral ischemia in rats. *Brain Res.* **580,** 197–204.

33. Yli-Hankala A., Edmonds H. L., Jr., Jiang Y. D., Higham H. E., and Zhang P. Y. (1997) Outcome effects of different protective hypothermia levels during cardiac arrest in rats. *Acta Anaesthesiol. Scand.* **41,** 511–515.

34. Kader A., Brisman M. H., Maraire N., Huh J. T., and Solomon R. A. (1992) The effect of mild hypothermia on permanent focal ischemia in the rat. *Neurosurgery* **31,** 1056–1060; discussion 1060–1061.

35. Karibe H., Zarow G. J., Graham S. H., and Weinstein P. R. (1994) Mild intraischemic hypothermia reduces postischemic hyperperfusion, delayed postischemic hypoperfusion, blood–brain barrier disruption, brain edema, and neuronal damage volume after temporary focal cerebral ischemia in rats. *J. Cereb. Blood Flow Metab.* **14,** 620–627.

36. Baker C. J., Onesti S. T., and Solomon R. A. (1992) Reduction by delayed hypothermia of cerebral infarction following middle cerebral artery occlusion in the rat: a time-course study. *J. Neurosurg.* **77,** 438–444.

37. Yanamoto H., Hong S. C., Soleau S., Kassell N. F., and Lee K. S. (1996) Mild postischemic hypothermia limits cerebral injury following transient focal ischemia in rat neocortex. *Brain Res.* **718,** 207–211.

38. Yanamoto H., Nagata I., Nakahara I., Tohnai N., Zhang Z., and Kikuchi H. (1999) Combination of intraischemic and postischemic hypothermia provides potent and persistent neuroprotection against temporary focal ischemia in rats. *Stroke* **30,** 2720–2726.

39. Huh P. W., Belayev L., Zhao W., Koch S., Busto R., and Ginsberg M. D. (2000) Comparative neuroprotective efficacy of prolonged moderate intraischemic and postischemic hypothermia in focal cerebral ischemia. *J. Neurosurg.* **92,** 91–99.

40. Maier C. M., Sun G. H., Kunis D., Yenari M. A., and Steinberg G. K. (2001) Delayed induction and long-term effects of mild hypothermia in a focal model of transient cerebral ischemia: neurological outcome and infarct size. *J. Neurosurg.* **94,** 90–96.

41. Steinberg G. K., Grant G., and Yoon E. (1995) Deliberate hypothermia. In *Intraoperative Neuroprotection* (Andrews R., ed.), Williams & Wilkins, Baltimore, pp. 65–84.

42. Todd M. M. and Warner D. S. (1992) A comfortable hypothesis reevaluated. Cerebral metabolic depression and brain protection during ischemia. *Anesthesiology* **76,** 161–164.

43. Nakashima K., Todd M. M., and Warner D. S. (1995) The relation between cerebral metabolic rate and ischemic depolarization. A comparison of the effects of hypothermia, pentobarbital, and isoflurane. *Anesthesiology* **82,** 1199–1208.

44. Kuluz J. W., Prado R., Chang J., Ginsberg M. D., Schleien C. L., and Busto R. (1993) Selective brain cooling increases cortical cerebral blood flow in rats. *Am. J. Physiol.* **265,** H824–827.

45. Sakamoto T. and Monafo W. W. (1989) Regional blood flow in the brain and spinal cord of hypothermic rats. *Am. J. Physiol.* **257,** H785–790.

46. Sick T. J., Tang R., and Pérez-Pinzón M. A. (1999) Cerebral blood flow does not mediate the effect of brain temperature on recovery of extracellular potassium ion activity after transient focal ischemia in the rat. *Brain Res.* **821,** 400–406.

47. Baldwin W. A., Kirsch J. R., Hurn P. D., Toung W. S., and Traystman R. J. (1991) Hypothermic cerebral reperfusion and recovery from ischemia. *Am. J. Physiol.* **261,** H774–781.

48. Lo E. H. and Steinberg G. K. (1992) Effects of hypothermia on evoked potentials, magnetic resonance imaging, and blood flow in focal ischemia in rabbits. *Stroke* **23,** 889–893.

49. Huang F. and Zhou L. (1998) Effect of mild hypothermia on the changes of cerebral blood flow, brain blood barrier and neuronal injuries following reperfusion of focal cerebral ischemia in rats. *Chin. Med. J. (Engl.)* **111,** 368–372.

50. Yanamoto H., Nagata I., Niitsu Y., et al. (2001) Prolonged mild hypothermia therapy protects the brain against permanent focal ischemia. *Stroke* **32,** 232–239.

51. Nagai S., Irikura K., Maruyama S., and Miyasaka Y. (1999) The significance of hypothermic acid-base management induced before ischemia in a rat model of transient middle cerebral artery occlusion. *Neurol. Res.* **21,** 204–208.

52. Kollmar R., Frietsch T., Georgiadis D., et al. (2002) Early effects of acid–base management during hypothermia on cerebral infarct volume, edema, and cerebral blood flow in acute focal cerebral ischemia in rats. *Anesthesiology* **97,** 868–874.

53. Baker A. J., Zornow M. H., Grafe M. R., et al. (1991) Hypothermia prevents ischemia-induced increases in hippocampal glycine concentrations in rabbits. *Stroke* **22,** 666–673.

54. Illievich U. M., Zornow M. H., Choi K. T., Strnat M. A., and Scheller M. S. (1994) Effects of hypothermia or anesthetics on hippocampal glutamate and glycine concentrations after repeated transient global cerebral ischemia. *Anesthesiology* **80,** 177–186.

55. Nakashima K. and Todd M. M. (1996) Effects of hypothermia on the rate of excitatory amino acid release after ischemic depolarization. *Stroke* **27,** 913–918.

56. Simpson R. E., Walter G. A., and Phillis J. W. (1991) The effects of hypothermia on amino acid neurotransmitter release from the cerebral cortex. *Neurosci. Lett.* **124,** 83–86.

57. Graham S. H., Shiraishi K., Panter S. S., Simon R. P., and Faden A. I. (1990) Changes in extracellular amino acid neurotransmitters produced by focal cerebral ischemia. *Neurosci. Lett.* **110,** 124–130.

58. Huang F. P., Zhou L. F., and Yang G. Y. (1998) Effects of mild hypothermia on the release of regional glutamate and glycine during extended transient focal cerebral ischemia in rats. *Neurochem. Res.* **23,** 991–996.

59. Baker C. J., Fiore A. J., Frazzini V. I., Choudhri T. F., Zubay G. P., and Solomon R. A. (1995) Intraischemic hypothermia decreases the release of glutamate in the cores of permanent focal cerebral infarcts. *Neurosurgery* **36**, 994–1001.
60. Nowak T. S. and Pulsinelli W. A. (1999) Delayed hypothermic protection after transient focal ischemia in spontaneously hypertensive rats. *Stroke* **30**, 246.
61. Xue D., Huang Z. G., Smith K. E., and Buchan A. M. (1992) Immediate or delayed mild hypothermia prevents focal cerebral infarction. *Brain Res.* **587**, 66–72.
62. Kawai N., Kawanishi M., Okauchi M., and Nagao S. (2001) Effects of hypothermia on thrombin-induced brain edema formation. *Brain Res.* **895**, 50–58.
63. Huang Z. G., Xue D., Preston E., Karbalai H., and Buchan A. M. (1999) Biphasic opening of the blood–brain barrier following transient focal ischemia: effects of hypothermia. *Can. J. Neurol Sci.* **26**, 298–304.
64. Kollmar R., Schabitz W. R., Heiland S., et al. (2002) Neuroprotective effect of delayed moderate hypothermia after focal cerebral ischemia: an MRI study. *Stroke* **33**, 1899–1904.
65. Mitani A. and Kataoka K. (1991) Critical levels of extracellular glutamate mediating gerbil hippocampal delayed neuronal death during hypothermia: brain microdialysis study. *Neuroscience* **42**, 661–670.
66. Mori K., Miyazaki M., Iwase H., and Maeda M. (2002) Temporal profile of changes in brain tissue extracellular space and extracellular ion (Na(+), K(+)) concentrations after cerebral ischemia and the effects of mild cerebral hypothermia. *J. Neurotrauma* **19**, 1261–1270.
67. Snider B. J., Gottron F. J., and Choi D. W. (1999) Apoptosis and necrosis in cerebrovascular disease. *Ann. NY Acad. Sci.* **893**, 243–253.
68. Kochanek P. M. and Hallenbeck J. M. (1992) Polymorphonuclear leukocytes and monocytes/macrophages in the pathogenesis of cerebral ischemia and stroke. *Stroke* **23**, 1367–1379.
69. Phillis J. W. (1994) A "radical" view of cerebral ischemic injury. *Prog. Neurobiol.* **42**, 441–448.
70. Imaizumi S., Kayama T., and Suzuki J. (1984) Chemiluminescence in hypoxic brain—the first report. Correlation between energy metabolism and free radical reaction. *Stroke* **15**, 1061–1065.
71. Kirsch J. R., Helfaer M. A., Lange D. G., and Traystman R. J. (1992) Evidence for free radical mechanisms of brain injury resulting from ischemia/reperfusion-induced events. *J. Neurotrauma* **9(Suppl. 1)**, S157–163.
72. Globus M. Y., Alonso O., Dietrich W. D., Busto R., and Ginsberg M. D. (1995) Glutamate release and free radical production following brain injury: effects of posttraumatic hypothermia. *J. Neurochem.* **65**, 1704–1711.
73. Kil H. Y., Zhang J., and Piantadosi C. A. (1996) Brain temperature alters hydroxyl radical production during cerebral ischemia/reperfusion in rats. *J. Cereb. Blood Flow Metab.* **16**, 100–106.
74. Lei B., Adachi N., and Arai T. (1997) The effect of hypothermia on H_2O_2 production during ischemia and reperfusion: a microdialysis study in the gerbil hippocampus. *Neurosci. Lett.* **222**, 91–94.
75. Wenisch C., Narzt E., Sessler D. I., et al. (1996) Mild intraoperative hypothermia reduces production of reactive oxygen intermediates by polymorphonuclear leukocytes. *Anesth. Analg.* **82**, 810–816.
76. Patel M., Day B. J., Crapo J. D., Fridovich I., and McNamara J. O. (1996) Requirement for superoxide in excitotoxic cell death. *Neuron* **16**, 345–355.

77. Karibe H., Chen S. F., Zarow G. J., et al. (1994) Mild intraischemic hypothermia suppresses consumption of endogenous antioxidants after temporary focal ischemia in rats. *Brain Res.* **649,** 12–18.

78. Liu X. H., Kato H., Nakata N., Kogure K., and Kato K. (1993) An immunohistochemical study of copper/zinc superoxide dismutase and manganese superoxide dismutase in rat hippocampus after transient cerebral ischemia. *Brain Res.* **625,** 29–37.

79. Matsuyama T., Michishita H., Nakamura H., et al. (1993) Induction of copper-zinc superoxide dismutase in gerbil hippocampus after ischemia. *J. Cereb. Blood Flow Metab.* **13,** 135–144.

80. Fukuhara T., Gotoh M., Kawauchi M., Asari S., and Ohmoto T. (1994) Superoxide scavenging activity in the extracellular space of the brain in forming edema. *Neurosurgery* **35,** 924–928; discussion 929.

81. Gonzalez-Scarano F. and Baltuch G. (1999) Microglia as mediators of inflammatory and degenerative diseases. *Annu. Rev. Neurosci.* **22,** 219–240.

82. Karabiyikoglu M., Han H. S., Yenari M. A., and Steinberg G. K. (2003) Attenuation of nNOS and iNOS expression by mild hypothermia after focal cerebral ischemia depends on when cooling begins. *J. Neurosurg.* **98,** 1271–1276.

83. Maier C., Tannous N., Steinberg G., and Chan P. (2001) Increased rate of hemorrhage in SOD2-deficient mice after transient focal cerebral ischemia: effect of mild hypothermia. *Neurology* **56,** A305.

84. Akins P. T., Liu P. K., and Hsu C. Y. (1996) Immediate early gene expression in response to cerebral ischemia. Friend or foe? *Stroke* **27,** 1682–1687.

85. Kamme F. and Wieloch T. (1996) The effect of hypothermia on protein synthesis and the expression of immediate early genes following transient cerebral ischemia. *Adv. Neurol.* **71,** 199–206.

86. Prakasa Babu P., Yoshida Y., Su M., Segura M., Kawamura S., and Yasui N. (2000) Immunohistochemical expression of Bcl-2, Bax and cytochrome c following focal cerebral ischemia and effect of hypothermia in rat. *Neurosci. Lett.* **291,** 196–200.

87. Yenari M. A., Iwayama S., Cheng D., et al. (2002) Mild hypothermia attenuates cytochrome c release but does not alter Bcl-2 expression or caspase activation after experimental stroke. *J. Cereb. Blood Flow Metab.* **22,** 29–38.

88. Xu L., Yenari M. A., Steinberg G. K., and Giffard R. G. (2002) Mild hypothermia reduces apoptosis of mouse neurons in vitro early in the cascade. *J. Cereb. Blood Flow Metab.* **22,** 21–28.

4

Hypothermic Protection in Traumatic Brain Injury

W. Dalton Dietrich, PhD,
and Miguel A. Pérez-Pinzón, PhD

INTRODUCTION

The beneficial effects of mild to moderate hypothermia in experimental models of traumatic brain injury (TBI) have been demonstrated in a large number of laboratories throughout the world (for review, *see* Dietrich, 1996 *[1]* and Gordon, 2001 *[2]*). Using TBI models of diffuse as well as focal injury, mild and moderate hypothermia have been reported to protect, both histopathologically and functionally. In contrast, posttraumatic hyperthermia worsens traumatic outcome *(3–5)*. Recently, these experimental findings have been supported by clinical data, in which treatment with hypothermia has improved outcome in stroke and trauma patients with severe brain injury *(6–8)*. Based on these data, a resurgence in the potential use of therapeutic hypothermia in experimental models of central nervous system (CNS) injury has occurred. The purpose of this chapter is to review experimental data obtained in animal models of brain trauma demonstrating the beneficial effects of mild to moderate hypothermia and to consider potential mechanisms underlying such hypothermic protection.

HISTOPATHOLOGICAL PROTECTION

Quantitative strategies to evaluate the effects of posttraumatic temperature patterns of neuronal vulnerability in models of TBI have been conducted in several laboratories. The effect of posttraumatic hypothermia on histopathological outcome was first evaluated in a model of moderate parasagittal fluid percussion (F-P) brain injury *(3)*. In that

From: *Hypothermia and Cerebral Ischemia: Mechanisms and Clinical Applications*
Edited by: C. M. Maier and G. K. Steinberg © Humana Press Inc., Totowa, NJ

study, brain temperature was selectively decreased to 30°C beginning 5 min after moderate trauma (1.7–2.2 atm) and maintained for a 3-h period. Three days later, contusion volume and frequency of damaged cortical neurons were compared in hypothermic vs normothermic (37.5°C) rats. Posttraumatic hypothermia significantly decreased contusion volume and reduced the frequency of damaged cortical neurons. In a controlled cortical impact model in rats, mild hypothermia (32–33°C) initiated 30 min before trauma and continued for 2 h after trauma significantly decreased contusion volume at 14 d (9). In contrast to the results reported with F-P injury, no significant effect on structural pathology, as reflected by cortical neurons or hippocampal cell survival, was reported with posttraumatic hypothermia (32°C/2 h) after cortical impact injury (10). Taken together, these findings from different TBI models (i.e., diffuse vs focal) emphasize the importance of the magnitude of TBI in determining whether structural protection can be observed with restricted periods of hypothermia.

The long-term effects of posttraumatic hypothermia have been evaluated in a parasagittal F-P model (11). Following normothermic TBI (2.0–2.3 atm), widespread atrophy of gray matter structures and enlargement of the lateral ventricle were reported at 2 mo following trauma. Importantly, posttraumatic hypothermia (30°C/3 h) significantly attenuated the degree of cortical atrophy and inhibited the ventricular enlargement. Using a similar model, Matsushita et al. (12) showed that posttraumatic hypothermia (33°C, 4-h duration) could significantly reduce contusion volumes as long as rewarming occurred slowly (120 min vs 15 min). Together, these experimental findings indicate that cerebral hypothermia alone following TBI is clearly a potent therapeutic approach to reducing neuronal damage in a variety of injury models.

Trauma-induced axonal injury (TAI) is an important feature of human TBI. Some investigations have reported that moderate hypothermia can also reduce the generation of traumatically induced axonal injury (6,13). In one study, moderate hypothermia (32°C/4 h) initiated 10 min or 25 min after injury significantly reduced the number of abnormally stained axonal profiles (6). A study by Koizumi and Povlishock (13) reported that posttraumatic hypothermia (32°C/1 h) initiated as late as 1 h after trauma significantly reduced the density of amyloid precursor protein (APP) immunoreactive damaged axons within the corticospinal tract. Together, these data indicate that posttraumatic hypothermia in two models of TBI provides substantial protection in terms of axonal injury. The finding that posttraumatic hypothermia protects against trauma-induced axonal injury would be expected to result in improved circuit function after TBI. It is important to note that, in severe TBI, the beneficial effects of hypothermia may be more limited. Indeed, a study by Brodhun et al. *(14)* showed that severe TBI caused by F-P and combined with temporary blood loss consistently produced traumatic axonal injury that could not be rescued by hypothermic treatment (32°C for 6 h, commenced 1 h postinjury).

BEHAVIORAL IMPROVEMENT WITH POSTTRAUMATIC HYPOTHERMIA

Although the histopathological assessment of the injured brain is considered to be an important endpoint for evaluating neuroprotective strategies, it is critical to determine whether histopathological protection also correlates with improved behavioral performance. Clifton et al. *(15)* first reported that hypothermia (30°C and 33°C) decreased mortality rates and improved beam-balance and beam-walking tasks, compared with normothermic rats (38°C) after midline F-P brain injury (2.1–2.25 atm). Subsequent studies by Lyeth et al. *(16)* reported behavioral protection by moderate hypothermia (30°C/1 h) initiated 15 min but not 30 min after midline moderate F-P injury in rats. This study indicated that the therapeutic window for moderate hypothermia might be relatively short after TBI in the rat. Other studies using the parasagittal F-P model demonstrated that posttraumatic hypothermia (30°C/3 h) begun 10 min following injury also improved both sensorimotor and cognitive function *(11)*. Recently, Markgraf et al. *(17)* demonstrated that when hypothermia was initiated immediately or 60 min after TBI, injured rats showed less edema and improved functional outcome. Delaying hypothermic treatment by 90 min or more did not reduce edema formation or improve neurological outcome. Cognitive deficits, including memory impairment, are commonly observed in humans suffering brain injury. Thus, the ability to improve cognitive function after TBI by hypothermic strategies appears to be an interesting direction in treating the brain-injured patient.

In clinical studies, posttraumatic hypothermia has also been reported to be beneficial *(7,18)*. Marion et al. *(18)* demonstrated that posttraumatic hypothermia (32–33°C/24 h) in patients with severe TBI and Glasgow Coma Scores of 5–7 on admission hastened neurologic recovery and may have improved outcome. These clinical findings are important in that they indicate that preclinical data are relevant to the clinical condition of TBI.

REWARMING PHASE

In addition to the degree and duration of cooling being critical factors in hypothermia treatment after TBI, rewarming conditions are of major consideration. In a study of transient forebrain ischemia, rapid rewarming failed to provide the neuroprotective effect of hypothermia that was observed with slow rewarming *(19)*. Similar findings have been recently obtained in a model of TBI with secondary hypoxia *(12)* and following TAI *(20)*. Importantly, gradual rewarming after controlled hypothermia has also been reported to produce axonal protection *(13)*. Thus, although the detrimental consequences of rapid postinjury warming in the clinical arena are routinely appreciated, the importance of rewarming conditions in experimental models of brain trauma require additional investigation.

POSTTRAUMATIC HYPERTHERMIA

Posttraumatic hyperthermia (>39°C), in contrast to hypothermia, has been shown in experimental models of TBI to worsen outcome. In one study, artificially elevating brain temperature to 39°C for a 3-h period, 24 h after moderate parasagittal F-P injury increased mortality, compared with normothermic rats *(1)*. Delayed hyperthermia also significantly increased contusion volume and increased the frequency of abnormal-appearing myelinated axons.

Many head-injured patients experience fever, and recent data indicate that bladder temperature and rectal temperature often underrepresent brain temperature after TBI, particularly when the patient is hypo- or hyperthermic *(21)*. In that study, brain temperature was usually greater than rectal or bladder temperature in adults with severe brain injury. In another study, the duration of fever was reported to be associated with poor outcome in patients with supratentorial hemorrhage *(5)*. Taken together, these experimental and clinical findings *(4,5)* indicate that fever should be aggressively treated when core temperature is mildly elevated above normal levels *(22,23)*.

MECHANISMS OF HYPOTHERMIC PROTECTION

The pathophysiology of TBI is complex, and many injury processes have been reported to be temperature sensitive. Indeed, the fact that relatively small variations in brain temperature can affect multiple cellular processes may account for the dramatic effects of temperature on variations in numerous animal models of brain injury. Whether future research can identify a single injury process or primary mechanism responsible for the effects of temperature on injury is unclear. Nevertheless, continued research into the understanding of temperature mechanisms should improve the treatment and care of TBI patients.

ION HOMEOSTASIS

Ion homeostasis is highly dependent on adequate provisions of ATP, which in turn is highly sensitive to different types of stress conditions in the CNS. Disturbances in ion homeostasis following acute brain injuries have been studied extensively *(24)*. Few studies have examined the effect of TBI on ion homeostasis, and thus the information on ionic fluxes following TBI is very scant. Walker et al. *(25)* suggested a breakdown of ion gradients and cell depolarization immediately following brain trauma. These findings were supported by Takahashi et al. *(26)* in a model of brain trauma, in which ion-selective microelectrodes were used. They showed a significant increase in extracellular potassium in the cortex. Increases in extracellular potassium were confirmed using the microdialysis technique *(27)*. Nilsson et al. *(28)* reported that compression contusion trauma produces a transient membrane depolarization associated with a pronounced cellular release of potassium and a massive calcium entry into intracellular compartments. They suggested that leaky membranes exposed to shear stress mediated ionic derangements.

To date, no study has reported a correlation between the neuroprotection afforded by hypothermia to improvements in ion homeostasis following TBI. Nevertheless, data have been reported correlating hypothermia and ion gradient derangements following cerebral ischemia. Foremost among the processes that might explain the temperature sensitivity of the brain to ischemia are energy metabolism and functions requiring high-energy use such as ion transport. It is well known that ischemia is accompanied within minutes by sudden, large shifts in the concentrations of most extracellular ion species (anoxic depolarization [AD]), suggesting ionic equilibration across cellular membranes *(24)*. In focal ischemia these changes are limited to regions of severely limited blood flow *(29)*. However, in regions surrounding the ischemic core, transient ionic disturbances occur that closely resemble cortical spreading depression (SD). The ionic changes associated with focal ischemic are important because they may contribute to brain infarction *(30,31)*.

There have been few reports on the effects of temperature on brain ion homeostasis after ischemia. However, there appears to be a consensus that hypothermia does not prevent AD associated with either global or focal ischemia, although it has been reported that the onset of AD may be delayed *(32–34)*. It has also been reported that mild hypothermia reduces the number of SD-like depolarizations associated with focal ischemia *(34)*. The frequency of SD-like depolarizations has been associated with the degree of damage after focal ischemia *(35,36)*. It is possible that the same occurs following TBI.

While there has been considerable interest in the ionic changes that occur during focal ischemia, little attention has been paid to disturbances associate with reperfusion. Most earlier investigations, for example, have shown that extracellular potassium ion activity recovers to or near preischemic levels on reperfusion *(29,37)*, suggesting normalization of potassium ion homeostasis. We have recently shown, however, that focal ischemia is accompanied by early secondary elevation of extracellular potassium ion activity that is dependent on brain temperature but not cerebral blood flow *(38)*.

EXCITOTOXICITY

In addition to slowing oxygen consumption, posttraumatic hypothermia has been shown to inhibit the rise in extracellular levels of excitatory amino acids and the production of hydroxyl radicals, compared with normothermic trauma *(39)*. In that study, the magnitude of glutamate release was correlated with the extent of hydroxyl radical production, raising the possibility that the two responses represented important mechanisms by which hypothermia confers protection following TBI. On the other hand, a clinical study by Soukup et al. *(40)* showed that patients with spontaneous brain hypothermia on admission (brain temperature < 36.0°C) showed significantly higher levels of glutamate as well as lactate, compared to all other patients, and had a worse outcome. The authors concluded that spontaneous brain hypothermia carries a poor prognosis, and is characterized by markedly abnormal brain metabolic indices.

MITOCHONDRIAL DYSFUNCTION

Mitochondrial dysfunction has been linked to the causes of metabolic impairment following TBI *(41)*. Xiong et al. *(42)* demonstrated that significant decreases in state 3 respiratory rates, respiratory control index (RCI), and P/O ratios occurred as early as 1 h and persisted for at least 14 d following TBI. These values could be restored if a calcium chelator (EGTA) was administered to the assay mixture. Those results suggested that TBI perturbs cellular calcium homeostasis, resulting in excessive calcium accumulation into mitochondria. This excessive calcium uptake into mitochondria can subsequently inhibit the electron transport chain for oxidative phosphorylation. Inhibition of the electron transport chain, in turn, can promote free radical formation. This has been supported by numerous studies on TBI, but Xiong et al. *(42)* demonstrated a direct link. They administered U-101033E, a novel antioxidant, following TBI. This antioxidant effectively restored normal mitochondrial function.

The role of mitochondria as a mediator of cell death has been supported by findings that cytochrome *c*, a proapoptotic molecule, is released from mitochondria following TBI *(43)*. This evidence is supported further by findings that cyclosporin A, an inhibitor of the permeability transition pore of mitochondria, which has been hypothesized as a key mechanism for the release of cytochrome *c*, is protective against cell death following TBI *(44–51)*. Furthermore, there is mounting evidence that various enzymatic pathways connected to mitochondrial function and cytochrome *c* release are activated following TBI *(52–56)*.

Despite all of the evidence the mitochondria are at the core of cell death/dysfunction following TBI, there is still no evidence that hypothermia is protective by ameliorating mitochondrial dysfunction.

EDEMA AND THE BLOOD-BRAIN BARRIER

The detrimental consequences of blood–brain barrier (BBB) dysfunction after TBI have also been reported to be reduced by hypothermia *(57)*. Alteration in BBB permeability may contribute to the detrimental effects of TBI through swelling or excitotoxic processes, as well as allowing abnormal passage of blood-borne exogenous neurotransmitters into the brain and influencing injury processes *(58)*.

GENE EXPRESSION AND CYTOKINE PRODUCTION

In addition to the neurotransmitter and hydroxyl radical consequences, postinjury temperature modification has been shown to affect the induction of immediate early genes/protooncogenes and influence upregulated cytokine expression. For example, hypothermia was reported to attenuate the normal increase in interleukin-1 RNA and nerve growth factor in traumatized rats *(59)*. Recent laboratory studies have shown that TBI produces a loss of cytoskeletal proteins, including neurofilaments, spectrin, and microtubule-associated protein-2 (MAP2). Importantly, Taft et al. *(60)* have shown that hypothermia attenuates the loss of hippocampal MAP2 following TBI. Thus, temperature modifications after injury may be affecting both extracellular and intracellular processes critical to neuronal survival.

NITRIC OXIDE

Recent studies have demonstrated the importance of nitric oxide (NO) in the pathophysiology of TBI. Wada and colleagues *(61)* reported that cortical constitutive NOS (cNOS) catalytic activity increases 5 min after TBI in the histopathologically damaged cerebral cortex, returned to control levels by 30 min, and was reduced at 1 and 7 d. In another study, inducible NOS (iNOS) activity was reported to be elevated at 3 and 7 d after TBI *(61)*. Because limited data are available concerning the effects of therapeutic hypothermia on NOS activity following TBI, a recent study by Chatzipanteli et al. *(62)* reported the effects of cooling on alteration in cNOS and iNOS activities following TBI. Importantly, posttraumatic hypothermia (30°C) decreased early cNOS activation and prevented the delayed induction of iNOS. Thus, temperature-dependent alteration in NOS activities may participate in the neuroprotective effects of posttraumatic hypothermia.

APOPTOSIS

The mechanism of delayed neuronal injury following TBI includes apoptosis *(63,64)*. Experimental data after cerebral hypoxic–ischemic injury indicate that moderate postinsult hypothermia (34°C) reduced the fraction of apoptotic cells but not cells undergoing necrosis *(65)*. In another study, intraischemic hypothermia reduced the number of transferase dUTP nick-end labeling (TUNEL)-positive cells after transient focal ischemia *(66)*. Thus, it will be important in future studies to determine whether hypothermia inhibits apoptotic neuronal cell death in models of TBI.

INFLAMMATION

Traumatic brain injury leads to inflammatory events that are believed to contribute to outcome through secondary injury mechanisms *(67,68)*.

Recent investigations have determined the effects of posttraumatic temperature modification on inflammatory responses following brain injury. In one study using the cortical impact model of TBI, polymorphonuclear leukocyte accumulation in the injured cortex was significantly depressed in rats maintained at 32°C vs 39°C *(69)*. Data from another laboratory have indicated that both posttraumatic hypothermia and hyperthermia significantly influence the inflammatory consequences of parasagittal F-P brain injury *(70)*. Thus, at 3 h and 3 d after TBI, hypothermia reduced myeloperoxidase (MPO) activity in injured brain regions, while posttraumatic hyperthermia (39°C) significantly elevated MPO activity compared with normothermic (37°C) rats. A recent study by Kinoshita et al. *(71)* also showed that posttraumatic temperature manipulations alter the cerebrovascular and inflammatory consequences of TBI: posttraumatic hypothermia reduced hemoglobin extravasation at 24 h post F-P, whereas hyperthermia increased it. The same group also showed that proinflammatory cytokine interleukin-1β (IL-1β) protein levels were reduced by posttraumatic hypothermia (33°C) treatment *(72)*. Taken together, these results indicate that temperature-dependent alterations in secondary inflammatory processes appear to be potential mechanisms by which posttraumatic temperature modifications may influence traumatic outcome.

SUMMARY

Based on experimental and clinical data, cerebral hypothermia appears to be a potent therapeutic approach to treating brain trauma. However, recent results from the Multicenter National Brain Injury Study: Hypothermia (NABIS: H) clinical trial appear to be disappointing, and more refinement of the clinical application of hypothermia is required *(73)*. Additional clinical trials are now required to evaluate systematically the beneficial effects of clinical hypothermia in different populations of brain-injured patients. In addition, experimental data regarding the beneficial effects of combination therapy are required to evaluate whether hypothermia plus pharmacotherapy may provide a better outcome. For example, mild postischemic hypothermia (33–39°C) combined with the antiinflammatory cytokine IL-10 has recently been reported to produce long-term protection of the CA1 hippocampus after transient global ischemia *(74)*. Hypothermia or IL-10 treatment alone did not protect chronically. In contrast, Kline et al. *(75)* showed that acute systemic administration of IL-10 suppressed the beneficial effects of hypothermia (32°C/3 h) following TBI. Finally, the continued search for pharmacologic agents that reduce core and brain temperature when given systemically is an exciting direction. The development of this class of drugs would allow emergency room staff to administer agents at early periods of brain trauma.

ACKNOWLEDGMENTS

This work was supported by Grant NS30291 from the National Institutes of Health and The Miami Project to Cure Paralysis. The authors thank Charlaine Rowlette for editorial assistance and manuscript preparation.

REFERENCES

1. Dietrich W. D. (1996) Nonpharmacological strategies: moderate hypothermia. In *Neurotrauma* (Narayan R. K., Wilberger J. E., and Povlishock J. T., eds.), McGraw-Hill, New York, pp. 1491–1506.
2. Gordon C. J. (2001) The therapeutic potential of regulated hypothermia. *Emerg. Med. J.* **18,** 81–89.
3. Dietrich W. D., Alonso O., Busto R., Globus M. Y., and Ginsberg M. D. (1994) Post-traumatic brain hypothermia reduces histopathological damage following concussive brain injury in the rat. *Acta Neuropathol.* **87,** 250–258.
4. Aldana P. P., Marquez J., Petrin D. S., Johns D., Dietrich W. D., and Villanueva P. A. (1998) Hyperthermia adversely affects outcome after moderate head injury. *J. Neurotrauma* **15,** 854.
5. Schwarz S., Hafner K., Aschoff A., and Schwab S. (2000) Incidence and prognostic significance of fever following intracerebral hemorrhage. *Neurology* **54,** 354–361.
6. Marion D. W. and White M. J. (1996) Treatment of experimental brain injury with moderate hypothermia and 21-aminosteroids. *J. Neurotrauma* **13,** 139–147.
7. Clifton G. L. (1995) Systemic hypothermia in treatment of severe brain injury: a review and update. *J. Neurotrauma* **12,** 923–927.
8. Schwab S., Schwarz S., Spranger M., Keller E., Bertram M., and Hacke W. (1998) Moderate hypothermia in the treatment of patients with severe middle cerebral artery infarction. *Stroke* **29,** 2461–2466.
9. Palmer A. M., Marion D. W., Botscheller M. L., and Redd E. E. (1993) Therapeutic hypothermia is cytoprotective without attenuating the traumatic brain injury-induced elevations in interstitial concentrations of aspartate and glutamate. *J. Neurotrauma* **10,** 363–372.
10. Dixon C. E., Markgraf C. G., Angileri F., et al. (1998) Protective effects of moderate hypothermia on behavioral deficits but not necrotic cavitation following cortical impact injury in the rat. *J. Neurotrauma* **15,** 95–103.
11. Bramlett H. M., Dietrich W. D., Green E. J., and Busto R. (1997) Chronic histopathological consequences of fluid-percussion brain injury in rats: effects of post-traumatic hypothermia. *Acta Neuropathol. (Berl.)* **93,** 190–199.

12. Matsushita Y., Bramlett H. M., Alonso O., and Dietrich W. D. (2001) Posttraumatic hypothermia is neuroprotective in a model of traumatic brain injury complicated by a secondary hypoxic insult. *Crit. Care Med.* **29,** 2060–2066.

13. Koizumi H. and Povlishock J. T. (1998) Posttraumatic hypothermia in the treatment of axonal damage in an animal model of traumatic axonal injury. *J. Neurosurg.* **89,** 303–309.

14. Brodhun M., Fritz H., Walter B., et al. (2001) Immunomorphological sequelae of severe brain injury induced by fluid-percussion in juvenile pigs—effects of mild hypothermia. *Acta Neuropathol. (Berl.)* **101,** 424–434.

15. Clifton G. L., Jiang J. Y., Lyeth B. G., Jenkins L. W., Hamm R. J., and Hayes R. L. (1991) Marked protection by moderate hypothermia after experimental traumatic brain injury. *J. Cereb. Blood Flow Metab.* **11,** 114–121.

16. Lyeth B. G., Jiang J. Y., and Liu S. (1993) Behavioral protection by moderate hypothermia initiated after experimental traumatic brain injury. *J. Neurotrauma* **10,** 57–64.

17. Markgraf C. G., Clifton G. L., and Moody M. R. (2001) Treatment window for hypothermia in brain injury. *J. Neurosurg.* **95,** 979–983.

18. Marion D. W., Penrod L. E., Kelsey S. F., et al. (1997) Treatment of traumatic brain injury with moderate hypothermia. *N. Engl. J. Med.* **336,** 540–546.

19. Nakamura T., Miyamoto O., Yamagami S., Hayashida Y., Itano T., and Nagao S. (1999) Influence of rewarming conditions after hypothermia in gerbils with transient forebrain ischemia. *J. Neurosurg.* **91,** 114–120.

20. Suehiro E., Singleton R. H., Stone J. R., and Povlishock J. T. (2001) The immunophilin ligand FK506 attenuates the axonal damage associated with rapid rewarming following posttraumatic hypothermia. *Exp. Neurol.* **172,** 199–210.

21. Henker R. A., Brown S. D., and Marion D. W. (1998) Comparison of brain temperature with bladder and rectal temperatures in adults with severe head injury. *Neurosurgery* **42,** 1071–1075.

22. Cairns C. J. and Andrews P. J. (2002) Management of hyperthermia in traumatic brain injury. *Curr. Opin. Crit. Care* **8,** 106–110.

23. Soukup J., Zauner A., Doppenberg E. M., et al. (2002) The importance of brain temperature in patients after severe head injury: relationship to intracranial pressure, cerebral perfusion pressure, cerebral blood flow, and outcome. *J. Neurotrauma* **19,** 559–571.

24. Hansen A. J. and Nedergaard M. (1988) Brain ion homeostasis in cerebral ischemia. *Neurochem. Pathol.* **9,** 195–209.

25. Walker A., Kollros J., and Case T. (1944) The physiological basis of concussion. *J. Neurosurg.* **1,** 103–116.

26. Takahashi H., Manaka S., and Sano K. (1981) Changes in extracellular potassium concentration in cortex and brain stem during the acute phase of experimental closed head injury. *J. Neurosurg.* **55,** 708–717.

27. Katayama Y., Becker D. P., Tamura T., and Hovda D. A. (1990) Massive increases in extracellular potassium and the indiscriminate release of glutamate following concussive brain injury. *J. Neurosurg.* **73,** 889–900.

28. Nilsson P., Hillered L., Olsson Y., Sheardown M. J., and Hansen A. J. (1993) Regional changes in interstitial K^+ and Ca^{2+} levels following cortical compression contusion trauma in rats. *J. Cereb. Blood Flow Metab.* **13,** 183–192.

29. Branston N. M., Strong A. J., and Symon L. (1977) Extracellular potassium activity, evoked potential and tissue blood flow. Relationships during progressive ischaemia in baboon cerebral cortex. *J. Neurol. Sci.* **32,** 305–321.

30. Betz A. L., Ennis S. R., and Schielke G. P. (1989) Blood–brain barrier sodium transport limits development of brain edema during partial ischemia in gerbils. *Stroke* **20,** 1253–1259.

31. Young W., Rappaport Z. H., Chalif D. J., and Flamm E. S. (1987) Regional brain sodium, potassium, and water changes in the rat middle cerebral artery occlusion model of ischemia. *Stroke* **18,** 751–759.

32. Astrup J., Skovsted P., Gjerris F., and Sorensen H. R. (1981) Increase in extracellular potassium in the brain during circulatory arrest: effects of hypothermia, lidocaine, and thiopental. *Anesthesiology* **55,** 256–262.

33. Lantos J., Temes G., and Torok B. (1986) Changes during ischaemia in extracellular potassium ion concentration of the brain under nitrous oxide or hexobarbital-sodium anaesthesia and moderate hypothermia. *Acta Physiol. Hung.* **67,** 141–153.

34. Chen Q., Chopp M., Bodzin G., and Chen H. (1993) Temperature modulation of cerebral depolarization during focal cerebral ischemia in rats: correlation with ischemic injury. *J. Cereb. Blood Flow Metab.* **13,** 389–394.

35. Busch E., Gyngell M. L., Eis M., Hoehn-Berlage M., and Hossmann K. A. (1996) Potassium-induced cortical spreading depressions during focal cerebral ischemia in rats: contribution to lesion growth assessed by diffusion-weighted NMR and biochemical imaging. *J. Cereb. Blood Flow Metab.* **16,** 1090–1099.

36. Nedergaard M. and Astrup J. (1986) Infarct rim: effect of hyperglycemia on direct current potential and [^{14}C]2-deoxyglucose phosphorylation. *J. Cereb. Blood Flow Metab.* **6,** 607–615.

37. Gido G., Kristian T., and Siesjo B. K. (1997) Extracellular potassium in a neocortical core area after transient focal ischemia. *Stroke* **28,** 206–210.

38. Sick T. J., Tang R., and Perez-Pinzon M. A. (1999) Cerebral blood flow does not mediate the effect of brain temperature on recovery of extracellular potassium ion activity after transient focal ischemia in the rat. *Brain Res.* **821,** 400–406.

39. Globus M. Y., Alonso O., Dietrich W. D., Busto R., and Ginsberg M. D. (1995) Glutamate release and free radical production following brain injury: effects of posttraumatic hypothermia. *J. Neurochem.* **65,** 1704–1711.

40. Soukup J., Zauner A., Doppenberg E. M., et al. (2002) Relationship between brain temperature, brain chemistry and oxygen delivery after severe human head injury: the effect of mild hypothermia. *Neurol. Res.* **24,** 161–168.

41. Frantseva M., Perez Velazquez J. L., Tonkikh A., Adamchik Y., and Carlen P. L. (2002) Neurotrauma/neurodegeneration and mitochondrial dysfunction. *Prog. Brain Res.* **137,** 171–176.

42. Xiong Y., Gu Q., Peterson P. L., Muizelaar J. P., and Lee C. P. (1997) Mitochondrial dysfunction and calcium perturbation induced by traumatic brain injury. *J. Neurotrauma* **14,** 23–34.

43. Morita-Fujimura Y., Fujimura M., Kawase M., Chen S. F., and Chan P. H. (1999) Release of mitochondrial cytochrome c and DNA fragmentation after cold injury-induced brain trauma in mice: possible role in neuronal apoptosis. *Neurosci. Lett.* **267,** 201–205.

44. Buki A., Okonkwo D. O., and Povlishock J. T. (1999) Postinjury cyclosporin A administration limits axonal damage and disconnection in traumatic brain injury. *J. Neurotrauma* **16,** 511–521.

45. Okonkwo D. O. and Povlishock J. T. (1999) An intrathecal bolus of cyclosporin A before injury preserves mitochondrial integrity and attenuates axonal disruption in traumatic brain injury. *J. Cereb. Blood Flow Metab.* **19,** 443–451.

46. Scheff S. W. and Sullivan P. G. (1999) Cyclosporin A significantly ameliorates cortical damage following experimental traumatic brain injury in rodents. *J. Neurotrauma* **16,** 783–792.

47. Sullivan P. G., Thompson M. B., and Scheff S. W. (1999) Cyclosporin A attenuates acute mitochondrial dysfunction following traumatic brain injury. *Exp. Neurol.* **160,** 226–234.

48. Sullivan P. G., Thompson M., and Scheff S. W. (2000) Continuous infusion of cyclosporin A postinjury significantly ameliorates cortical damage following traumatic brain injury. *Exp. Neurol.* **161,** 631–637.

49. Albensi B. C., Sullivan P. G., Thompson M. B., Scheff S. W., and Mattson M. P. (2000) Cyclosporin ameliorates traumatic brain-injury-induced alterations of hippocampal synaptic plasticity. *Exp. Neurol.* **162,** 385–389.

50. Alessandri B., Rice A. C., Levasseur J., DeFord M., Hamm R. J., and Bullock M. R. (2002) Cyclosporin A improves brain tissue oxygen consumption and learning/memory performance after lateral fluid percussion injury in rats. *J. Neurotrauma* **19,** 829–841.

51. Lifshitz J., Friberg H., Neumar R. W., et al. (2003) Structural and functional damage sustained by mitochondria after traumatic brain injury in the rat: evidence for differentially sensitive populations in the cortex and hippocampus. *J. Cereb. Blood Flow Metab.* **23,** 219–231.

52. Knoblach S. M., Nikolaeva M., Huang X., et al. (2002) Multiple caspases are activated after traumatic brain injury: evidence for involvement in functional outcome. *J. Neurotrauma* **19,** 1155–1170.

53. Sullivan P. G., Keller J. N., Bussen W. L., and Scheff S. W. (2002) Cytochrome c release and caspase activation after traumatic brain injury. *Brain Res.* **949,** 88–96.

54. Harris L. K., Black R. T., Golden K. M., Reeves T. M., Povlishock J. T., and Phillips L. L. (2001) Traumatic brain injury-induced changes in gene expression and functional activity of mitochondrial cytochrome C oxidase. *J. Neurotrauma* **18,** 993–1009.

55. Yakovlev A. G. and Faden A. I. (2001) Caspase-dependent apoptotic pathways in CNS injury. *Mol. Neurobiol.* **24,** 131–144.

56. Lewen A., Fujimura M., Sugawara T., Matz P., Copin J. C., and Chan P. H. (2001) Oxidative stress-dependent release of mitochondrial cytochrome c after traumatic brain injury. *J. Cereb. Blood Flow Metab.* **21,** 914–920.

57. Jiang J. Y., Lyeth B. G., Kapasi M. Z., Jenkins L. W., and Povlishock J. T. (1992) Moderate hypothermia reduces blood–brain barrier disruption following traumatic brain injury in the rat. *Acta Neuropathol.* **84,** 495–500.

58. Lo E. H., Wang X., and Cuzner M. L. (2002) Extracellular proteolysis in brain injury and inflammation: role for plasminogen activators and matrix metalloproteinases. *J. Neurosci. Res.* **69,** 1–9.

59. Goss J. R., Styren S. D., Miller P. D., et al. (1995) Hypothermia attenuates the normal increase in interleukin 1 beta RNA and nerve growth factor following traumatic brain injury in the rat. *J. Neurotrauma* **12,** 159–167.

60. Taft W. C., Yang K., Dixon C. E., Clifton G. L., and Hayes R. L. (1993) Hypothermia attenuates the loss of hippocampal microtubule-associated protein 2 (MAP2) following traumatic brain injury. *J. Cereb. Blood Flow Metab.* **13,** 796–802.

61. Wada K., Chatzipanteli K., Kraydieh S., Busto R., and Dietrich W. D. (1998) Inducible nitric oxide synthase expression after traumatic brain injury and neuroprotection with aminoguanidine treatment in rats. *Neurosurgery* **43,** 1427–1436.

62. Chatzipanteli K., Wada K., Busto R., and Dietrich W. D. (1999) Effects of moderate hypothermia on constitutive and inducible nitric oxide synthase activities after traumatic brain injury in the rat. *J. Neurochem.* **72,** 2047–2052.

63. Rink A., Fung K. M., Trojanowski J. Q., Lee V. M., Neugebauer E., and McIntosh T. K. (1995) Evidence of apoptotic cell death after experimental traumatic brain injury in the rat. *Am. J. Pathol.* **147,** 1575–1583.

64. Conti A. C., Raghupathi R., Trojanowski J. Q., and McIntosh T. K. (1998) Experimental brain injury induces regionally distinct apoptosis during the acute and delayed post-traumatic period. *J. Neurosci.* **18,** 5663–5672.

65. Edwards A. D., Yue X., Squier M. V., et al. (1995) Specific inhibition of apoptosis after cerebral hypoxia-ischaemia by moderate post-insult hypothermia. *Biochem. Biophys. Res. Commun.* **217,** 1193–1199.

66. Toyoda T., Suzuki S., Kassell N. F., and Lee K. S. (1996) Intraischemic hypothermia attenuates neutrophil infiltration in the rat neocortex after focal ischemia-reperfusion injury. *Neurosurgery* **39,** 1200–1205.

67. Kettenmann H. (2002) Cellular components of neuroinflammation—an introduction. *Ernst Schering Res. Found. Workshop,* 1–9.

68. Morganti-Kossmann M. C., Rancan M., Stahel P. F., and Kossmann T. (2002) Inflammatory response in acute traumatic brain injury: a double-edged sword. *Curr. Opin. Crit. Care* **8,** 101–105.

69. Whalen M. J., Carlos T. M., Clark R. S., et al. (1997) The relationship between brain temperature and neutrophil accumulation after traumatic brain injury in rats. *Acta Neurochir. Suppl.* **70,** 260–261.

70. Chatzipanteli K., Alonso O. F., Kraydieh S., and Dietrich W. D. (2000) Importance of posttraumatic hypothermia and hyperthermia on the inflammatory response after fluid percussion brain injury: biochemical and immunocytochemical studies. *J. Cereb. Blood Flow Metab.* **20,** 531–542.

71. Kinoshita K., Chatzipanteli K., Alonso O. F., Howard M., and Dietrich W. D. (2002) The effect of brain temperature on hemoglobin extravasation after traumatic brain injury. *J. Neurosurg.* **97,** 945–953.

72. Kinoshita K., Chatzipanteli K., Vitarbo E., Truettner J. S., Alonso O. F., and Dietrich W. D. (2002) Interleukin-1beta messenger ribonucleic acid and protein levels after fluid-percussion brain injury in rats: importance of injury severity and brain temperature. *Neurosurgery* **51,** 195–203; discussion 203.

73. Clifton G. L., Miller E. R., Choi S. C., et al. (2001) Lack of effect of induction of hypothermia after acute brain injury. *N. Engl. J. Med.* **344,** 556–563.

74. Dietrich W. D., Busto R., and Bethea J. R. (1999) Postischemic hypothermia and IL-10 treatment provide long-lasting neuroprotection of CA1 hippocampus following transient global ischemia in rats. *Exp. Neurol.* **158,** 444–450.

75. Kline A. E., Bolinger B. D., Kochanek P. M., et al. (2002) Acute systemic administration of interleukin-10 suppresses the beneficial effects of moderate hypothermia following traumatic brain injury in rats. *Brain Res.* **937,** 22–31.

5

Postischemic Hypothermia Provides Long-Term Neuroprotection in Rodents

Frederick Colbourne, PhD,
and Dale Corbett, PhD

INTRODUCTION

Researchers in the field of cerebral ischemia traditionally rely on histological measures of brain injury to assess potential neuroprotectants such as hypothermia. In fact, cell counting procedures and infarct volume measurements are often the only endpoint used following global and focal cerebral ischemia, respectively. Furthermore, investigators commonly used short survival times (e.g., 1 d for focal ischemia, 7 d for global ischemia), as these were initially thought to encompass the time during which injury matured *(1–3)*. Several key studies in the past decade indicate that the maturation of ischemic injury is not fixed, but can be delayed considerably. Accordingly, the long-term histological benefit is yet unknown for most neuroprotectants. The lack of functional assessment in most studies raises further concerns about the true efficacy *(4)*.

Hypothermia is the most thoroughly investigated neuroprotectant for experimental cerebral ischemia. Hypothermia induced during ischemia provides substantial and lasting benefit (histological and functional) *(5– 8)*. However, at first glance, results with delayed cooling appear contradictory *(9)*. Several studies even suggest that postischemic hypothermia does not convey lasting protection. It is our view that such controversy largely stems from the use of ineffective or even harmful bouts of hypothermia and that recent failures to find persistent benefit are simply because cooling was not maintained for a sufficient period. Thus, the purpose of this chapter is to highlight recent studies that show

From: *Hypothermia and Cerebral Ischemia: Mechanisms and Clinical Applications*
Edited by: C. M. Maier and G. K. Steinberg © Humana Press Inc., Totowa, NJ

persistent/permanent functional and histological benefit with delayed postischemic hypothermia.

KEY STUDIES OF DELAYED HYPOTHERMIA IN RODENT GLOBAL CEREBRAL ISCHEMIA MODELS

Although studies of postischemic hypothermia date back to the 1950s, the recent work in rodents illustrates most of the important points. These studies, with few exceptions, examined hippocampal CA1 injury which, when untreated, was thought to mature over 24–72 h *(2,3)*. The first rodent experiments to show cellular protection with postischemic hypothermia were by Busto et al. *(10)* and Boris-Möller et al. *(11)*. The rat two-vessel occlusion model (2-VO, bilateral carotid artery occlusion + systemic hypotension) was used in both studies and hypothermia was induced immediately after ischemia. Busto et al. reduced CA1 loss at a 3-d survival with 3 h of cooling (30°C) while Boris-Möller et al. reduced damage to CA1, cortex, and striatum (7-d survival) with 2 h of 27°C hypothermia. Subsequently, other reports showed that a brief ($\leq$ 8 h) postischemic cooling (ranged between 27 and 34°C) reduced CA1 injury in rats *(12–14)* and gerbils *(15–17)* even when intervention was delayed for hours.

Several studies using brief hypothermia have not found evidence of CA1 protection *(18–22)*. However, such discordant findings are easily explained by a mismatch between the duration of hypothermia and the severity of the ischemic insult. For example, Chopp et al. *(12)* found that 2 h of postischemic hypothermia reduced CA1 loss against 8 but not 12 min of ischemia in rats. Similarly, other experiments indicate that the duration of hypothermia is critical *(14,17)*, as very brief cooling (e.g., 0.5 h) was ineffective while somewhat longer durations were (e.g., 5 h) protective, perhaps only transiently.

A study by Dietrich et al. *(23)* found that 3 h of immediate postischemic hypothermia (30°C) reduced CA1 loss at short (i.e., 3 and 7 d) but not long survival times (2 mo) after 10 min 2-VO ischemia in rats. Because all of the aforementioned studies (e.g., refs. *10–14*) used short survival times, it was argued that postischemic hypothermia was, by itself, of no long-term benefit. Other work has confirmed the ephemeral nature of CA1 protection afforded by brief hypothermia *(24)*. Likewise, a slow maturation of CA1 neuronal loss occurs following short duration (e.g., 5 min) 4-VO (vertebral cauterization + bilateral carotid artery occlusion) ischemia *(25)*. In the 4-VO model the α-amino-3-hydroxy-

5-methyl-4-isoxazolepropionic acid (AMPA) antagonist 2,3-dihydroxy-6-nitro-7-sulfamoylbenzo(F)quinoxaline (NBQX) and the N-type calcium antagonist SNX-111 were found to delay rather than prevent CA1 neuronal death *(25)*. Taken together, these data strongly argue for the use of long-term survival times in all efficacy studies.

More recent studies have shown long-term protection with extended duration hypothermia induced following global ischemia in the gerbil *(26,27)* and rat *(28)*. The discrepancy between these studies and previous failures *(23,24)* to document persistent neuroprotection is attributable to the greater efficacy of protracted hypothermia. In one study gerbils were subjected to 3 or 5 min of normothermic forebrain ischemia followed 1 h later by 12 h of 32°C hypothermia. Notably, 3–5 min of normothermic bilateral carotid artery occlusion in the gerbil will, by itself, produce dense forebrain ischemia with resultant CA1 injury similar to 10 or more minutes of 2-VO or 4-VO ischemia in rats. While 12 h of hypothermia was not very efficacious against a 5-min insult, cooling was almost totally protective in CA1 after a 10- and 30-d survival time against the 3-min occlusion. Thus, as Chopp et al. *(12)* found, hypothermia was more efficacious against the milder insult. What is more important, this study highlighted the importance of using protracted durations of postischemic hypothermia, as 24 h of hypothermia (91% CA1 survival) was more than six *times* more effective (30-d survival) than a 12-h duration (<15% CA1 cell survival) against a 5-min occlusion that otherwise would have destroyed ≈ 99% of CA1 cells. Follow-up studies have confirmed that 1- *(26)*, 6- *(28,29)*, and even 12- *(9)* h delayed hypothermic interventions in adult gerbils can provide chronic CA1 protection (1- to 2-mo survival times). In addition, 1-h delayed hypothermia was persistently neuroprotective in aged gerbils *(30)*. Finally, these results in gerbil are similar to recent findings in the rat 4-VO model where 6-h delayed hypothermia (32°C and later 34°C each for 24 h) provided robust CA1 neuroprotection (86% CA1 cell survival against a severe 10-min occlusion at a 28-d survival time *(31)*. Untreated, this insult resulted in 99% CA1 loss. Likewise, Coimbra et al. *(32)* found long-term protection with 7 h of mild hypothermia (2-h intervention delay) against milder insult in the 2-VO model.

We have investigated the ultrastructural morphology of ischemic CA1 cell death and the effects of delayed postischemic hypothermia *(33)*. Although CA1 cell death was largely attenuated by postischemic hypothermia, some CA1 neurons nonetheless died, and the ultrastructural features of this death were typical of necrosis (e.g., membrane breaks). Surprisingly, while most neurons protected by hypothermia were ultrastructurally normal, a few had sublethal signs of injury (e.g., organelle dilations) while others had evidence of extensive mitochondrial injury (i.e., abundant mitochondrial autolysosomes). Thus, although delayed hypothermia treatment is efficacious, some neurons are not perfectly preserved. It may be these neurons that eventually succumb and contribute to residual/partial functional impairments (e.g., see refs. *26,28*).

In addition to robust CA1 neuroprotection (**Fig. 1**), postischemic hypothermia also markedly reduces ischemic functional impairments. The first study *(27)* to show this examined exploratory behavior in an open field test on d 3, 7, and 10 following ischemia in gerbils. Subsequent studies *(26,28)* confirm that postischemic hypothermia can largely attenuate exploratory deficits. Likewise, ischemia-induced working memory impairments *(34–36)*, due to CA1 loss, have been significantly attenuated with 1- *(26)* and even 6- *(28)* h delayed hypothermia (**Fig. 2**). Results form a recent study of forebrain ischemia *(37)* showed that some of the hypothermia-salvaged CA1 neurons are susceptible to delayed, normally sublethal, transient ischemic attacks (TIAs) following hypothermic neuroprotection, yet many hypothermia-salvaged neurons are resilient to TIAs. In that study, hypothermia treatment was delayed for 12 h. Behavioral testing did not distinguish between gerbils with or without TIA, but did reveal deficits in the normothermic ischemic gerbils and protection in the hypothermic ischemic gerbils. This is important because it suggests that the clinical efficacy of treatments administered after cerebral ischemia might be undone by insults that would otherwise remain untreated. In that study, the authors also suggest that aggressive rehabilitation therapies may need to be delayed to avoid losing some previously saved tissue.

In summary, the severity of ischemia has a critical impact on the amount of neuroprotection obtained with postischemic hypothermia *(12,27)*. Brief hypothermic periods (e.g., <5 h) are not very efficacious and only delay cell death. Prolonged bouts (e.g., 24–48 h) of hypothermia

---

Fig. 1. *(opposite page)* CA1 sector photomicrographs (×400, hematoxylin and eosin staining) from a normal young adult gerbil (A), an untreated ischemic (5 min bilateral carotid artery occlusion) young gerbil (B), and from hypothermia (1-h delay, 24-h at 32°C)-treated ischemic gerbil (C = 4-mo-old; D = 18-mo-old). Hypothermic CA1 neuroprotection was robust in both young (27) and old *(30)* gerbils.

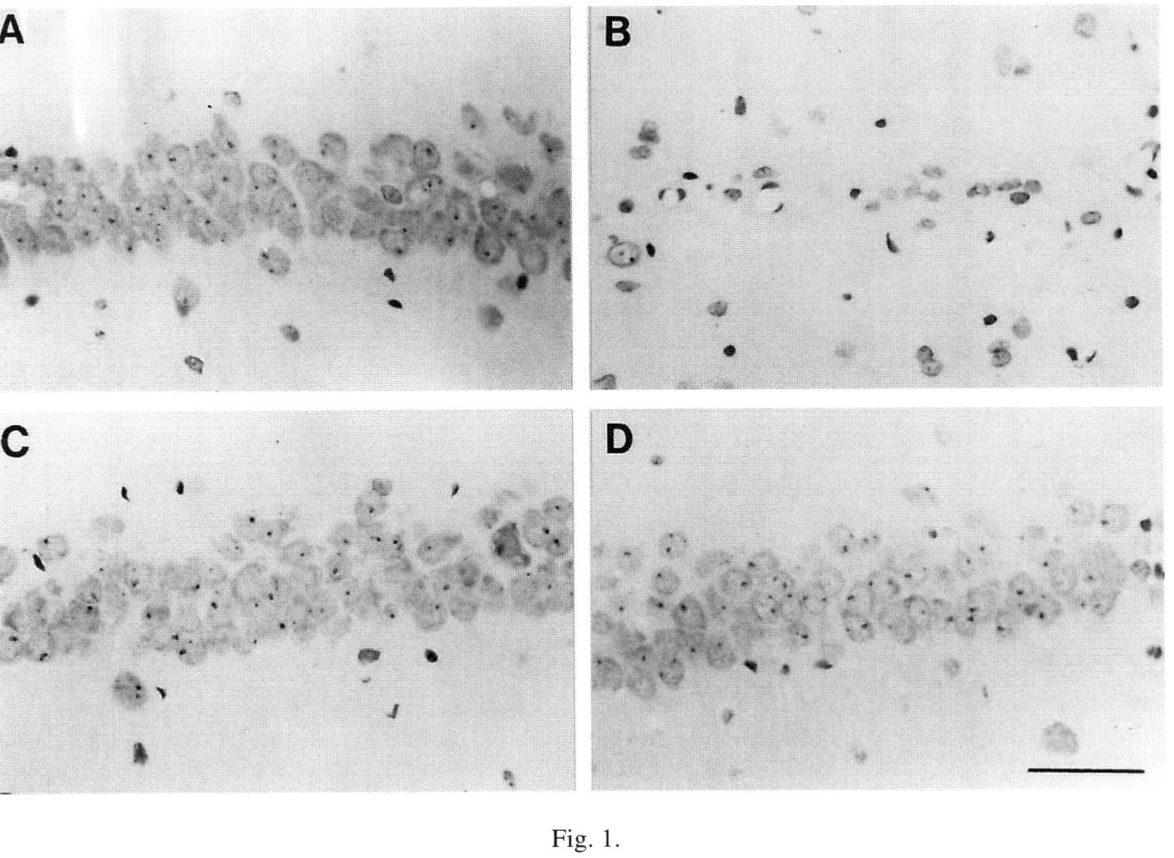

Fig. 1.

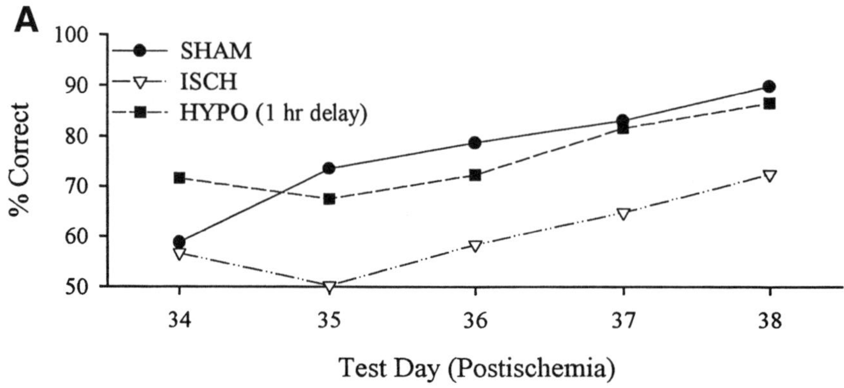

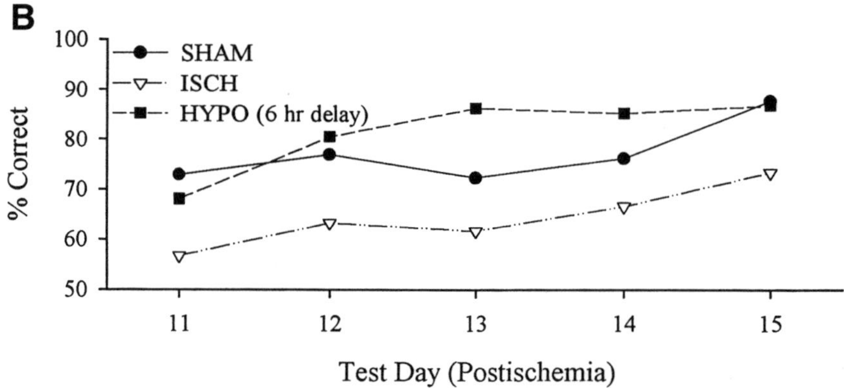

Fig. 2. T-maze performance (% correct) in gerbils trained on a win-shift strategy to find sunflower seeds (50% is chance level). Gerbils were subjected to sham operation (SHAM) or 5 min of normothermic ischemia with (HYPO) or without delayed hypothermic treatment (ISCH). In (A) the HYPO group was cooled for 1 d at 32°C starting at 1 h after ischemia *(26)*, while in (B) the HYPO gerbils were cooled (32°C + 34°C each for 1 d) starting 6 h after ischemia *(28)*. Untreated ischemia resulted in significantly more working memory errors (lower % correct) than SHAM animals, while the HYPO groups were well protected and this generally reflected CA1 cell count data.

convey lasting neuroprotection as first shown in the gerbil *(27)*. Milder hypothermic levels (34°C) are less protective than 32°C cooling *(26)*. Finally, the therapeutic window critically depends on the duration of hypothermia (e.g., compare reference *[26]* with *[28,33]* and compare reference *[10]* with *[31]*).

STUDIES OF DELAYED POSTISCHEMIC HYPOTHERMIA IN CANINE GLOBAL CEREBRAL ISCHEMIA MODELS

The aforementioned findings in rodents mirror results observed in dogs subjected to cardiac arrest with subsequent postischemic mild hypothermia of 1- to 12-h duration *(38–44)*. For example, a 12-h period of 34°C hypothermia with hemodilution and elevated blood pressure reduced brain injury (e.g., hippocampus, neocortex, basal ganglia) and lessened functional deficits after cardiac arrest. However, in all of these studies the survival time was 4 d or less, and thus it has yet to be proven that postischemic hypothermia can permanently reduce ischemic brain injury in the dog. Based on the rodent literature, it would be useful to investigate more protracted bouts of mild hypothermia and assess long-term outcome in this intensive cardiac arrest model in the dog.

KEY STUDIES OF DELAYED HYPOTHERMIA IN FOCAL CEREBRAL ISCHEMIA

There are numerous studies that show that intraischemic hypothermia reduces focal ischemic injury (e.g., from a middle cerebral artery occlusion [MCAO]). More clinically relevant are the experiments that find a reduction in infarct volume when cooling is instituted near the end of or after MCAO in adult rats with brief *(45–51)* and prolonged *(52,53)* postischemic hypothermia. Some of these studies also illustrate the importance of treatment duration *(47,48,51,52)*. Because infarction may develop slowly following untreated *(54,55)* or treated *(56)* MCAO, it is noteworthy that two studies assessed infarction at a 1-wk survival *(45,46)* while another assessed infarction at 2 mo *(53)*. In the latter study, we subjected rats to 30 min of MCA occlusion by an intraluminal insertion of a suture at a systemic blood pressure of 60 mmHg, which markedly aggravates injury *(57)*. Two days of 34°C hypothermia was then instituted, starting 30 min into reperfusion. Hypothermia produced a striking reduction in cortical infarction at a 2-mo survival time while the near-total loss of striatal tissue was marginally but significantly attenuated.

Studies in neonatal rats support these findings. For instance, Sirimanne et al. *(58)* persistently (21-d survival) reduced infarction in 21-d-old rats with 72 h of immediate postischemic mild hypothermia. Gunn et al. *(59)* reduced cortical infarction (5-d survival) in fetal sheep with the use of 72 h of mild *in utero* hypothermia induced 90 min after the start of ischemia. As in global ischemia, these data contrast with brief postischemic hypothermia (e.g., 3 h), which failed to reduce hypoxic–ischemic injury in rat pups *(60)*.

Contrary to later findings, early studies of prolonged hypothermia in dogs, cats, and monkeys indicate that prolonged cooling is detrimental. In one study, 48 h of 29°C hypothermia was induced (under paralysis and diazepam sedation) starting 30 min into permanent MCA occlusion in Java monkeys *(61)*. All five monkeys died and this was significantly worse than following untreated ischemia (historical control group). Similarly, poor outcomes were found in MCA occluded and normal monkeys and cats *(62)* and in normal dogs *(63)* subjected to prolonged 29°C hypothermia. The lethality of rewarming was perhaps due to cardiovascular complications. These results contrast with the observation in rats and gerbils that prolonged mild hypothermia is safe and without any obvious pathological effect on various organs *(29)*. Likewise, Safar et al. *(44)* safely cooled dogs to 34°C for 12 h following cardiac arrest. Finally, there are the favorable results from some clinical trials of prolonged mild (i.e., 32–34°C) hypothermia in traumatic brain injury *(64–71)*. The most likely reason for the early negative findings in cats, monkeys and dogs apparently relate to the degree of hypothermia, as systemic side effects are more common when temperature is lowered below 30°C. Accordingly, studies in animal models *(26,27,31)* and humans *(64–71)* have maintained temperature above 30°C.

In summary, the data in focal ischemia suggest that mild hypothermia is beneficial while moderate cooling is detrimental. Clearly, the optimal pattern of hypothermia (depth and duration) is yet unknown and our current knowledge lags far behind that for global ischemia. Accordingly, the relatively short therapeutic window observed (i.e., 30 min after reperfusion *[47]*), which is an impediment to clinical investigation, may have grossly underestimated the true value of prolonged postischemic hypothermia. Thus, if the situation following focal ischemia is similar to global ischemia, then more prolonged periods of hypothermia may yield a substantially wider window of opportunity. Future studies should examine these possibilities, and also include assessment of functional outcomes.

CONCLUSIONS

Research into the beneficial effects of delayed hypothermia on ischemic injury was renewed largely as a result of the positive findings in rodent models of global cerebral ischemia in which the data prove that prolonged mild hypothermia can persistently reduce ischemic CA1 injury and attenuate functional deficits. Although data in focal cerebral ischemia are comparable, the limited number of studies does not yet allow firm conclusions as to maximal efficacy. Studies are in progress to address these issues. If further promising experimental and clinical (for head injury) results are found, then clinical trials of mild hypothermia for stroke and cardiac arrest encephalopathy will hopefully ensue. Regardless, the large number of publications that illustrate the profound influence of altered postischemic temperature (both hypothermia and hyperthermia; *see* refs. *8* and *9* for review) warrants the widespread adoption of careful temperature control in experimental studies and in the clinic. Finally, additional mechanistic studies into the beneficial actions of hypothermia might generate more selective and effective treatments for acute stroke.

REFERENCES

1. Garcia J. H., Yoshida Y., Chen H., et al. (1993) Progression from ischemic injury to infarct following middle cerebral artery occlusion in the rat. *Am. J. Pathol.* **142,** 623–635.
2. Kirino T. (1982) Delayed neuronal death in the gerbil hippocampus following ischemia. *Brain Res.* **239,** 57–69.
3. Pulsinelli W. A., Brierley J. B., and Plum F. (1982) Temporal profile of neuronal damage in a model of transient forebrain ischemia. *Ann. Neurol.* **11,** 491–498.
4. Corbett D. and Nurse S. (1998) The problem of assessing effective neuroprotection in experimental cerebral ischemia. *Prog. Neurobiol.* **54,** 531–548.
5. Ginsberg M. D., Sternau L. L., Globus M. Y., Dietrich W. D., and Busto R. (1992) Therapeutic modulation of brain temperature: relevance to ischemic brain injury. *Cerebrovasc. Brain Metab. Rev.* **4,** 189–225.
6. Maher J. and Hachinski V. (1993) Hypothermia as a potential treatment for cerebral ischemia. *Cerebrovasc. Brain Metab. Rev.* **5,** 277–300.
7. Dietrich W. D., Busto R., Globus M. Y., and Ginsberg M. D. (1996) Brain damage and temperature: cellular and molecular mechanisms. *Adv. Neurol.* **71,** 177–194.
8. Busto R. and Ginsberg M. D. (1998) The influence of altered brain temperature in cerebral ischemia. In *Cerebrovascular Disease: Pathophysiology, Diagnosis, and Management* (Ginsberg M. D. and Bogousslavsky J., eds.), Blackwell Science, Malden, pp. 287–307.
9. Colbourne F., Sutherland G., and Corbett D. (1997) Postischemic hypothermia. A critical appraisal with implications for clinical treatment. *Mol. Neurobiol.* **14,** 171–201.
10. Busto R., Dietrich W. D., Globus M. Y., and Ginsberg M. D. (1989) Postischemic moderate hypothermia inhibits CA1 hippocampal ischemic neuronal injury. *Neurosci. Lett.* **101,** 299–304.

11. Boris-Möller F., Smith M.-L., and Siesjo B. K. (1989) Effect of hypothermia on ischemic brain damage: a comparison between preischemic and postischemic cooling. *Neurosci. Res. Comm.* **5,** 87–94.
12. Chopp M., Chen H., Dereski M. O., and Garcia J. H. (1991) Mild hypothermic intervention after graded ischemic stress in rats. *Stroke* **22,** 37–43.
13. Coimbra C. and Wieloch T. (1992) Hypothermia ameliorates neuronal survival when induced 2 hours after ischaemia in the rat. *Acta Physiol. Scand.* **146,** 543–544.
14. Coimbra C. and Wieloch T. (1994) Moderate hypothermia mitigates neuronal damage in the rat brain when initiated several hours following transient cerebral ischemia. *Acta Neuropathol.* **87,** 325–331.
15. Buchan A. and Pulsinelli W. A. (1990) Hypothermia but not the *N*-methyl-D-aspartate antagonist, MK-801, attenuates neuronal damage in gerbils subjected to transient global ischemia. *J. Neurosci.* **10,** 311–316.
16. Coimbra C. G. and Cavalheiro E. A. (1990) Protective effect of short-term postischemic hypothermia on the gerbil brain. *Braz. J. Med. Biol. Res.* **23,** 605–611.
17. Carroll M. and Beek O. (1992) Protection against hippocampal CA1 cell loss by post-ischemic hypothermia is dependent on delay of initiation and duration. *Metab. Brain Dis.* **7,** 45–50.
18. Welsh F. A. and Harris V. A. (1991) Postischemic hypothermia fails to reduce ischemic injury in gerbil hippocampus. *J. Cereb. Blood Flow Metab.* **11,** 617–620.
19. Chen H., Chopp M., Vande Linde A. M., Dereski M. O., Garcia J. H., and Welch K. M. (1992) The effects of post-ischemic hypothermia on the neuronal injury and brain metabolism after forebrain ischemia in the rat. *J. Neurol. Sci.* **107,** 191–198.
20. Iwai T., Niwa M., Yamada H., Nozaki M., and Tsurumi K. (1993) Hypothermic prevention of the hippocampal damage following ischemia in Mongolian gerbils comparison between intraischemic and brief postischemic hypothermia. *Life Sci.* **52,** 1031–1038.
21. Hara A., Yoshimi N., Mori H., et al. (1995) Hypothermic prevention of nuclear DNA fragmentation in gerbil hippocampus following transient forebrain ischemia. *Neurol. Res.* **17,** 461–464.
22. Xiao F., Safar P., and Radovsky A. (1998) Mild protective and resuscitative hypothermia for asphyxial cardiac arrest in rats. *Am. J. Emerg. Med.* **16,** 17–25.
23. Dietrich W. D., Busto R., Alonso O., Globus M. Y., and Ginsberg M. D. (1993) Intraischemic but not postischemic brain hypothermia protects chronically following global forebrain ischemia in rats. *J. Cereb. Blood Flow Metab.* **13,** 541–549.
24. Dietrich W. D., Lin B., Globus M. Y., Green E. J., Ginsberg M. D., and Busto R. (1995) Effect of delayed MK-801 (dizocilpine) treatment with or without immediate postischemic hypothermia on chronic neuronal survival after global forebrain ischemia in rats. *J. Cereb. Blood Flow Metab.* **15,** 960–968.
25. Colbourne F., Li H., Buchan A. M., and Clemens J. A. (1999) Continuing postischemic neuronal death in CA1: influence of ischemia duration and cytoprotective doses of NBQX and SNX-111 in rats. *Stroke* **30,** 662–668.
26. Colbourne F. and Corbett D. (1995) Delayed postischemic hypothermia: a six month survival study using behavioral and histological assessments of neuroprotection. *J. Neurosci.* **15,** 7250–7260.
27. Colbourne F. and Corbett D. (1994) Delayed and prolonged post-ischemic hypothermia is neuroprotective in the gerbil. *Brain Res.* **654,** 265–272.
28. Colbourne F., Auer R. N., and Sutherland G. R. (1998) Characterization of postischemic behavioral deficits in gerbils with and without hypothermic neuroprotection. *Brain Res.* **803,** 69–78.

29. Colbourne F., Auer R. N., and Sutherland G. R. (1998) Behavioral testing does not exacerbate ischemic CA1 damage in gerbils. *Stroke* **29,** 1967–1970; discussion 1971.
30. Corbett D., Nurse S., and Colbourne F. (1997) Hypothermic neuroprotection. A global ischemia study using 18- to 20-month-old gerbils. *Stroke* **28,** 2238–2242; discussion 2243.
31. Colbourne F., Li H., and Buchan A. M. (1999) Indefatigable CA1 sector neuroprotection with mild hypothermia induced 6 hours after severe forebrain ischemia in rats. *J. Cereb. Blood Flow Metab.* **19,** 742–749.
32. Coimbra C., Drake M., Boris-Moller F., and Wieloch T. (1996) Long-lasting neuroprotective effect of postischemic hypothermia and treatment with an anti-inflammatory/antipyretic drug. Evidence for chronic encephalopathic processes following ischemia. *Stroke* **27,** 1578–1585.
33. Colbourne F., Sutherland G., and Auer R. N. (1997) New features of delayed neuronal death in gerbils treated with prolonged postischemic hypothermia. *Soc. Neurosci. Abstr.* **23,** 1917.
34. Volpe B. T., Waczek B., and Davis H. P. (1988) Modified T-maze training demonstrates dissociated memory loss in rats with ischemic hippocampal injury. *Behav. Brain Res.* **27,** 259–268.
35. Volpe B. T., Davis H. P., Towle A., and Dunlap W. P. (1992) Loss of hippocampal CA1 pyramidal neurons correlates with memory impairment in rats with ischemic or neurotoxin lesions. *Behav. Neurosci.* **106,** 457–464.
36. Babcock A. M. and Graham-Goodwin H. (1997) Importance of preoperative training and maze difficulty in task performance following hippocampal damage in the gerbil. *Brain Res. Bull.* **42,** 415–419.
37. De Bow S. B. and Colbourne F. (2003) Delayed transient ischemic attacks kill some CA1 neurons previously salvaged with postischemic hypothermia: neuroprotection undone. *Brain Res.* **959,** 50–57.
38. Leonov Y., Sterz F., Safar P., and Radovsky A. (1990) Moderate hypothermia after cardiac arrest of 17 minutes in dogs. Effect on cerebral and cardiac outcome. *Stroke* **21,** 1600–1606.
39. Leonov Y., Sterz F., Safar P., et al. (1990) Mild cerebral hypothermia during and after cardiac arrest improves neurologic outcome in dogs. *J. Cereb. Blood Flow Metab.* **10,** 57–70.
40. Baldwin W. A., Kirsch J. R., Hurn P. D., Toung W. S., and Traystman R. J. (1991) Hypothermic cerebral reperfusion and recovery from ischemia. *Am. J. Physiol.* **261,** H774–781.
41. Safar P. and Sterz F. (1991) Mild hypothermic cardiopulmonary resuscitation. *Crit. Care Med.* **19,** 1217.
42. Weinrauch V., Safar P., Tisherman S., Kuboyama K., and Radovsky A. (1992) Beneficial effect of mild hypothermia and detrimental effect of deep hypothermia after cardiac arrest in dogs. *Stroke* **23,** 1454–1462.
43. Kuboyama K., Safar P., Radovsky A., Tisherman S. A., Stezoski S. W., and Alexander H. (1993) Delay in cooling negates the beneficial effect of mild resuscitative cerebral hypothermia after cardiac arrest in dogs: a prospective, randomized study. *Crit. Care Med.* **21,** 1348–1358.
44. Safar P., Xiao F., Radovsky A., et al. (1996) Improved cerebral resuscitation from cardiac arrest in dogs with mild hypothermia plus blood flow promotion. *Stroke* **27,** 105–113.

45. Zhang R. L., Chopp M., Chen H., Garcia J. H., and Zhang Z. G. (1993) Postischemic (1 hour) hypothermia significantly reduces ischemic cell damage in rats subjected to 2 hours of middle cerebral artery occlusion. *Stroke* **24,** 1235–1240.

46. Zhang Z. G., Chopp M., and Chen H. (1993) Duration dependent post-ischemic hypothermia alleviates cortical damage after transient middle cerebral artery occlusion in the rat. *J. Neurol. Sci.* **117,** 240–244.

47. Markarian G. Z., Lee J. H., Stein D. J., and Hong S. C. (1996) Mild hypothermia: therapeutic window after experimental cerebral ischemia. *Neurosurgery* **38,** 542–550; discussion 551.

48. Maier C. M., Ahern K., Cheng M. L., Lee J. E., Yenari M. A., and Steinberg G. K. (1998) Optimal depth and duration of mild hypothermia in a focal model of transient cerebral ischemia: effects on neurologic outcome, infarct size, apoptosis, and inflammation. *Stroke* **29,** 2171–2180.

49. Maier C. M., Sun G. H., Kunis D., Yenari M. A., and Steinberg G. K. (2001) Delayed induction and long-term effects of mild hypothermia in a focal model of transient cerebral ischemia: neurological outcome and infarct size. *J. Neurosurg.* **94,** 90–96.

50. Kollmar R., Schabitz W. R., Heiland S., et al. (2002) Neuroprotective effect of delayed moderate hypothermia after focal cerebral ischemia: an MRI study. *Stroke* **33,** 1899–1904.

51. Yanamoto H., Nagata I., Niitsu Y., et al. (2001) Prolonged mild hypothermia therapy protects the brain against permanent focal ischemia. *Stroke* **32,** 232–239.

52. Yanamoto H., Hong S. C., Soleau S., Kassell N. F., and Lee K. S. (1996) Mild postischemic hypothermia limits cerebral injury following transient focal ischemia in rat neocortex. *Brain Res.* **718,** 207–211.

53. Corbett D., Hamilton M., and Colbourne F. (2000) Persistent neuroprotection with prolonged postischemic hypothermia in adult rats subjected to transient middle cerebral artery occlusion. *Exp. Neurol.* **163,** 200–206.

54. Du C., Hu R., Csernansky C. A., Hsu C. Y., and Choi D. W. (1996) Very delayed infarction after mild focal cerebral ischemia: a role for apoptosis? *J. Cereb. Blood Flow Metab.* **16,** 195–201.

55. Endres M., Namura S., Shimizu-Sasamata M., et al. (1998) Attenuation of delayed neuronal death after mild focal ischemia in mice by inhibition of the caspase family. *J. Cereb. Blood Flow Metab.* **18,** 238–247.

56. Valtysson J., Hillered L., Andine P., Hagberg H., and Persson L. (1994) Neuro-pathological endpoints in experimental stroke pharmacotherapy: the importance of both early and late evaluation. *Acta Neurochir.* **129,** 58–63.

57. Zhu C. Z. and Auer R. N. (1995) Graded hypotension and MCA occlusion duration: effect in transient focal ischemia. *J. Cereb. Blood Flow Metab.* **15,** 980–988.

58. Sirimanne E. S., Blumberg R. M., Bossano D., et al. (1996) The effect of prolonged modification of cerebral temperature on outcome after hypoxic–ischemic brain injury in the infant rat. *Pediatr. Res.* **39,** 591–597.

59. Gunn A. J., Gunn T. R., de Haan H. H., Williams C. E., and Gluckman P. D. (1997) Dramatic neuronal rescue with prolonged selective head cooling after ischemia in fetal lambs. *J. Clin. Invest.* **99,** 248–256.

60. Yager J., Towfighi J., and Vannucci R. C. (1993) Influence of mild hypothermia on hypoxic-ischemic brain damage in the immature rat. *Pediatr. Res.* **34,** 525–529.

61. Michenfelder J. D. and Milde J. H. (1977) Failure of prolonged hypocapnia, hypothermia, or hypertension to favorably alter acute stroke in primates. *Stroke* **8,** 87–91.

62. Steen P. A., Soule E. H., and Michenfelder J. D. (1979) Detrimental effect of prolonged hypothermia in cats and monkeys with and without regional cerebral ischemia. *Stroke* **10,** 522–529.

63. Steen P. A., Milde J. H., and Michenfelder J. D. (1980) The detrimental effects of prolonged hypothermia and rewarming in the dog. *Anesthesiology* **52,** 224–230.

64. Clifton G. L. (1995) Systemic hypothermia in treatment of severe brain injury: a review and update. *J. Neurotrauma* **12,** 923–927.

65. Marion D. W., Obrist W. D., Carlier P. M., Penrod L. E., and Darby J. M. (1993) The use of moderate therapeutic hypothermia for patients with severe head injuries: a preliminary report. *J. Neurosurg.* **79,** 354–362.

66. Marion D. W., Penrod L. E., Kelsey S. F., et al. (1997) Treatment of traumatic brain injury with moderate hypothermia. *N. Engl. J. Med.* **336,** 540–546.

67. Shiozaki T., Sugimoto H., Taneda M., et al. (1993) Effect of mild hypothermia on uncontrollable intracranial hypertension after severe head injury. *J. Neurosurg.* **79,** 363–368.

68. Clifton G. L., Allen S., Berry J., and Koch S. M. (1992) Systemic hypothermia in treatment of brain injury. *J. Neurotrauma* **9(Suppl 2),** S487–495.

69. Piepgras A., Roth H., Schurer L., et al. (1998) Rapid active internal core cooling for induction of moderate hypothermia in head injury by use of an extracorporeal heat exchanger. *Neurosurgery* **42,** 311–317; discussion 317–318.

70. Shiozaki T., Sugimoto H., Taneda M., et al. (1998) Selection of severely head injured patients for mild hypothermia therapy. *J. Neurosurg.* **89,** 206–211.

71. Tateishi A., Soejima Y., Taira Y., et al. (1998) Feasibility of the titration method of mild hypothermia in severely head-injured patients with intracranial hypertension. *Neurosurgery* **42,** 1065–1069; discussion 1069–1070.

6

Combination Therapy With Hypothermia and Pharmaceuticals for the Treatment of Acute Cerebral Ischemia

David C. Tong, MD,
and Midori A. Yenari, MD

INTRODUCTION

Although the use of hypothermia alone in acute ischemic stroke shows substantial promise, the possibility of using it in combination with other neuroprotective treatments has only recently been studied in experimental models. The desired effect of combination therapy is to enhance the effectiveness of each individual neuroprotective modality. However, although the existence of synergistic effects from combination treatment makes great hypothetical sense, several potential pitfalls must be considered if combined therapy is ever to be implemented effectively. In this chapter, we explore the potential advantages of combining hypothermia with other neuroprotective treatment modalities, as well as discuss the potential drawbacks of such combined treatments. In addition, we identify areas that require further investigation before such combined therapy can be evaluated for effectiveness in humans, as well as consider possible clinical trial designs necessary to evaluate appropriately such combined treatments.

RATIONALE

There are many potential advantages to the use of hypothermia in combination with other neuroprotective agents. It is assumed that by

From: *Hypothermia and Cerebral Ischemia: Mechanisms and Clinical Applications*
Edited by: C. M. Maier and G. K. Steinberg © Humana Press Inc., Totowa, NJ

affecting more than one part of the ischemic cascade, there may be an additive or perhaps even a compound effect on the efficacy of neuroprotection. Because it is not a pharmaceutical per se, it is believed that the use of hypothermia would not adversely interact with other simultaneous neurological treatments.

The specific choice of treatments to be used in combination with hypothermia could be based on a variety of different approaches. First, there could be a direct synergistic effect between hypothermia and the other proposed treatment modality, presumably as a result of a complementary mode of action. For example, combining hypothermia with thrombolytic therapy might be an appropriate pairing in which the hypothermia prolongs the therapeutic window for subsequent definitive reperfusion. Similarly, hypothermia could be used just after thrombolysis, to prevent reperfusion induced injury and prolonging the viability of injured but not irreversibly damaged tissue.

Another possibility is using hypothermia in combination with a second neuroprotective agent such a glutamate receptor antagonist. In this scenario, the goal would be to create a compound effect, particularly if the alternative treatment had a mode of action that is enhanced by the neuroprotective mechanism of hypothermia. Certainly this strategy makes sense, as hypothermia reduces cerebral glutamate accumulation. However, the precise mechanism of hypothermic neuroprotection is unknown, and may involve a variety of factors. Thus, it may be more appropriate to base treatment on a lack of potential adverse interactions and other such practical aspects as the ability to administer safely the two treatments together, rather than on a theoretical mechanism of action only. These concerns indicate a need for very rigorous preclinical testing of any potential combination treatment before proceeding to further definitive human trials.

In addition, any proposed treatment with other agent(s) in conjunction with hypothermia will require very careful scrutiny of efficacy in preclinical models because of the marked benefit of hypothermia alone reported in many experimental studies. The addition of the alternative agent(s) must result in a clear-cut additional benefit compared with hypothermia treatment alone. Moreover, as previously discussed, it would be helpful to prove in both clinical and preclinical studies that each agent individually has some degree of benefit, as neither hypothermia nor neuroprotective pharmaceuticals have yet been definitively proven to be beneficial in clinical studies of acute stroke treatment.

Table 1
Potential Barriers to Combination Hypothermia
and Neuroprotective Treatment in Acute Ischemic Stroke

Shivering
Patient discomfort from cooling
Slow onset
Metabolic effects of hypothermia on neuroprotective drug pharmacokinetics
Increased complexity of treatment
Cost

POTENTIAL PITFALLS (TABLE 1)

What are the potential pitfalls of combining hypothermia with other treatment modalities? Perhaps the most important is the possibility that there will be some adverse interaction between the combined treatments. This is not a minor concern, as it is well known that many pharmaceutical agents exhibit adverse effects when used in combination with other agents. Many of these adverse effects can be serious if not life threatening. In fact, this problem with drug interactions is a major reason why many pharmaceutical treatments are not used in clinical practice.

For hypothermia, one major possible difficulty involves the effect of low temperature on metabolism and enzyme activity. Many pharmaceutical agents have reduced biological activity at lower temperature compared with higher temperature. The thrombolytic activity of recombinant tissue plasminogen activator (rt-PA), for example, is clearly temperature dependent, with decreased activity at lower temperature (1). Thus, the assumption that hypothermia will not have an adverse effect on other treatment agents cannot be presumed. Hypothermia is also known to reduce the activity of inflammatory and antiinfectious biological processes. This could potentially result in increased susceptibility to infection. This possibility is of particular concern because infections are a major cause of morbidity in stroke patients (2). Therefore, combination therapy with hypothermia and antiinflammatory agents could potentially worsen outcome.

Similarly, hypothermia has known effects on cardiac rhythm, electrolyte balance, and metabolism, all of which could be enhanced when combined with pharmaceutical agents such as calcium or other ion channel blockers. Thus, as with all possible treatments, there is the potential not only for improvement, but also significant harm if an inappropriate combination is employed.

In addition, there is the added complexity of finding the optimal dose of neuroprotective and hypothermia treatment that will result in the optimal degree of neural protection. Because of the possibility of treatment interactions, significant preclinical testing will be necessary to identify the most clinically feasible and neurologically potent therapeutic regimen. This may be quite difficult, as the translation of preclinical research to human subjects is inexact. Added testing in phase I (safety) and phase II (dose escalation) human trials will be necessary, with a special emphasis on possible adverse interactions between the treatments.

EXPERIMENTAL EVIDENCE

What is the evidence that hypothermia plus other potential neuroprotective therapies actually does improve outcome compared with individual neuroprotective agents? Surprisingly, there are few preclinical and no human studies that have examined this issue. The main reason for this lack of study likely stems from the added complexity necessary for a combined treatment study, and the desire by most researchers to identify individual agents with neuroprotective properties first before proceeding to evaluate combination treatments. However, a handful of experimental treatment studies have been performed using hypothermia in conjunction with other neuroprotective agents, with surprisingly mixed results.

TRANSIENT ISCHEMIA MODELS

A small number of investigators have studied the possibility of combination neuroprotection and hypothermia in experimental models. Most of these studies have involved transient global ischemia models in which hypothermia is combined with other neuroprotectants, such as a glutamate antagonist. Dietrich et al. *(3)*, for example, demonstrated significantly increased neuroprotection in a global model of transient (10 min) forebrain ischemia when the neuroprotective agent MK-801 was combined with 3 h of postischemic hypothermia. At 2-mo follow-up, animals receiving the combined treatment exhibited greater CA1 neural protection compared with animals treated with either agent separately. Surprisingly, the prolonged neuroprotective effect was evident even though the MK-801 was administered only at late intervals (3–7 d) after ischemia onset, suggesting that acute postischemic hypothermia of even relatively brief duration (3 h) can extend the therapeutic window for neuroprotective treatment. Similar effects have been described when combining hypothermia with other *N*-methyl-D-aspartate (NMDA) receptor antagonists such as dextromethorphan *(4)*, and the competitive NMDA antagonist CGS-19755 (Selfotel) *(5)*. Of interest, in both of these other studies, the neuroprotective agent was administered several days after the acute insult, yet still provided enhanced neuroprotection compared with either placebo or each agent separately. In addition, these effects were observed on both behavioral as well as histopathological measures, suggesting a clinically important benefit to combination treatment.

The neuroprotective effects of other compounds have also been demonstrated to be enhanced when combined with hypothermia. Guan et al. *(6)* evaluated the efficacy of hypothermia in combination with insulin-like growth factor (IGF) using a modified Levine hypoxic–ischemic model (right carotid ligation plus 10 min of hypoxia in neonatal animals). In this study, the use of hypothermia resulted in a significant extension of the therapeutic time window. Recovery in a cool vs a warm environment (23 C vs 31 C) extended the effectiveness of IGF-1 by up to 4 h.

Similarly, Schmid-Elsaesser et al. *(7)* reported a synergistic effect of hypothermia when added to therapy with either tirilizad or magnesium (Mg). In this study, rats were subjected to transient ischemia of 90 min duration using a suture occlusion model. Hypothermia was administered intraischemically and animals were rewarmed simultaneous with reperfusion. Subjects were treated with various combinations of the three agents, in a systematic fashion. A stepwise increase in the reduction in infarct volume was observed between Tirilizad + Mg, hypothermia alone, and hypothermia + tirilizad + Mg in combination.

However, not all combination treatment strategies have clearly demonstrated an enhanced effect from combination treatment. Ogilvy et al. *(8)*, for example, compared mild hypothermia, hypertensive treatment, and mannitol individually and in combination in a rabbit model of temporary focal ischemia (2-h occlusion, 4-h reperfusion). Although the infarcts in the "triple" therapy group were generally smaller than in the monotherapy groups, the difference did not reach statistical significance. In another study, when hypothermia was combined with the free radical scavenger *N-tert*-butyl-α-pheylnitrone (PBN), no significant additional improvement in outcome compared with either treatment alone was found *(9)*. Similarly, no additional neuroprotection was observed by barbiturate-induced burst suppression under mild hypothermic conditions in rats subjected to 90 min of MCAO *(10)*.

OTHER EXPERIMENTAL MODELS

The effect of hypothermia in combination with thrombolytics has also been evaluated in only a few experimental studies. Meden et al. *(11)* studied differences in thrombolytic effectiveness in a rat embolic stroke model. In this study, 2 h of intraischemic hypothermia was administered with or without thrombolytic therapy. Thrombolysis was initiated at 2 h after ischemia onset. The investigators found that both hypothermia and thrombolysis significantly reduced infarct volume, but they could not demonstrate any added benefit of thrombolysis over hypothermia alone. A recent study by Wang et al. *(12)* used a focal embolic brain ischemia model to study the effects of minocycline, an antiinflammatory agent, alone or in combination with mild hypothermia (34–35°C started 1 h after embolization, 2-h duration). The results showed that both minocycline and the hypothermia–minocycline combination reduced infarct volume significantly, but no additive effect was observed.

No preclinical studies of neuroprotectives plus hypothermia in permanent occlusion stroke models without thrombolysis have been reported. This is of particular importance because these permanent ischemia models may better simulate the events that occur clinically in the vast majority of stroke patients who do not receive reperfusion therapy with a thrombolytic agent. Such studies will be necessary before proceeding with clinical trials in stroke patients.

Kahveci et al. *(13)* compared the cerebral protective effects of two known protective anesthetics, isoflurane and propofol, in combination with hypothermia (33–34°C) after traumatic brain injury (TBI). In that study, the authors found that propofol anesthesia plus hypothermia following TBI was better than the isoflurane–hypothermia combination because it reduced intracranial pressure and increased cerebral perfusion pressure under those conditions.

FUTURE DIRECTIONS

As can be seen from this review, most of the evidence suggesting a benefit to combination treatment has been performed in models of transient global ischemia. These models are generally considered to simulate hypoxic ischemic injury such as that seen following cardiac arrest rather than the prolonged focal ischemia usually associated with acute ischemic stroke. Only one thrombolytic study has been reported, and it

Table 2
Preclinical Experimental Criteria
for Hypothermia Combination Treatment in Acute Stroke

Evidence of protection greater than that provided by each individual treatment alone

Delay neuroprotective treatment–hypothermia by a minimum time interval (preferably 30 min or more) after ischemia onset

Sustained neuroprotection at prolonged (weeks/months) time point

Efficacy in multiple models of ischemia, particularly permanent ischemia models

Extensive analysis of pharmacokinetics and physiologic changes and side effects of combination treatment

Simple treatment protocol

did not detect an added benefit to thrombolysis compared with hypothermia alone. Thus, the evidence supporting the use of hypothermia in combination with other treatment modalities remains very limited.

Although the experimental evidence supporting the use of hypothermia in combination with other neuroprotective agents at this point is small and somewhat conflicting, there is enough theoretical and hypothetical promise to justify further exploration *(14)*. Future studies will need to provide convincing evidence of a synergistic effect of hypothermia with other ischemic stroke therapies. These studies will require the assessment of combination treatment strategies in many different stroke models to prove that the results are robust (**Table 2**). In particular, studies will need to be done in permanent ischemia paradigms, as this model appears to reflect more accurately the situation that is believed to occur in most humans suffering from an acute cerebral infarction. Additional studies will also be needed to characterize precisely the therapeutic windows for combination treatment as well as ensure the safety of these combined treatment protocols. These latter studies will be particularly important if hypothermia is used in conjunction with biologicals such as thrombolytics that use enzymes that may have a reduced metabolic rate with cooling. Other pharmacological agents may have even greater alterations in pharmacokinetics with cooling as a result of reduced metabolism or other hypothermic induced metabolic effects.

In addition, the significant technical obstacles associated with hypothermic treatment such as patient shivering and increased patient sus-

Table 3
Clinical Trial Design Considerations
for Hypothermic Combination Treatment in Acute Ischemic Stroke

Randomized blinded design
Short latency to treatment (unless otherwise indicated from preclinical data)
Administration of treatment in a way most similar to that used in the most
    effective preclinical models
Sufficient sample size to detect clinically significant benefit
Simple treatment regimen
Adequate monitoring of drug safety

ceptibility to infection itself must be overcome. While these problems can certainly be solved, the feasibility of hypothermic treatment in clinical practice remains unclear. Moreover, in this financially sensitive time, the cost of these treatments will need to be carefully assessed, particularly if the resources required for combination treatment are high.

CLINICAL TRIAL CONSIDERATIONS FOR COMBINATION TREATMENT (TABLE 3)

Assuming such preclinical studies did show such beneficial effects to combination treatment, how would a clinical trial of such combination treatment be designed? Because hypothermia is not an easily blinded treatment, special care will be needed to ensure the avoidance of bias. This might include use of separate blinded evaluators of neurological outcome unrelated to the patients' care. Inclusion criteria for the trial should also ensure that patients are neither too severely disabled, nor too mild affected neurologically, to avoid ceiling and floor effects.

Aside from these randomization and blinding issues, other important factors will be time interval to treatment, length of treatment, mode of treatment administration, and sufficient safeguards to patient safety based on the known side effects of hypothermic therapy in conjunction with the other agent. This information should also be available based on the results of preclinical studies.

While a specific protocol for a combination hypothermia plus neuroprotective treatment trial cannot be detailed here, in general, a short latency to treatment, adequate length of treatment (presumably identified by preclinical studies), and close monitoring for side effects, particularly infections, electrolyte changes, and patient discomfort, will be necessary. In addition, a simple method of treatment administration and monitoring of the effects of hypothermia on drug pharmacokinetics will be desirable. Finally, ethical concerns will also require that an "active" control be used. This means that the combination treatment will be used in comparison against a single (presumably previously established) agent alone. This requirement will necessitate an increase in sample size, as the effectiveness of combined treatment will presumably be less when compared with an active treatment than with a placebo.

CONCLUSIONS

It is clear from this discussion that although there is significant potential for the use of hypothermia in combination with additional neuroprotective agents, it is premature to consider this a viable option in the near future. Moreover, there are no adequate data on the safety of such combination therapy. In fact, there is some evidence suggesting that hypothermia could result in such adverse effects as reduced thrombolytic efficacy and increased susceptibility to infectious complications.

Nevertheless, the possibility of combining hypothermia with other types of neuroprotection or thrombolysis is intriguing, and certainly deserves future study. However, if this treatment is ever to impact clinical practice, it is essential that appropriate preclinical studies be conducted. In particular, the rigorous evaluation of these combinations in a variety of ischemic models that most closely simulate the pathophysiology of acute ischemic stroke, is needed. Only after such extensive testing should the possibility of combination therapy be subsequently evaluated in randomized clinical trials.

REFERENCES

1. Yenari M. A., Palmer J. T., Bracci P. M., and Steinberg G. K. (1995) Thrombolysis with tissue plasminogen activator (tPA) is temperature dependent. *Thromb. Res.* **77,** 475–481.
2. Brott T. and Hacke W. (1998) General treatment of acute ischemic stroke. In *Cerebrovascular Disease Pathophysiology, Diagnosis and Management* (Ginsberg M. D. and Bogousslavsky J., eds.), Blackwell Science, Malden, pp. 1864–1878.
3. Dietrich W. D., Lin B., Globus M. Y., Green E. J., Ginsberg M. D., and Busto R. (1995) Effect of delayed MK-801 (dizocilpine) treatment with or without immediate postischemic hypothermia on chronic neuronal survival after global forebrain ischemia in rats. *J. Cereb. Blood Flow Metab.* **15,** 960–968.

4. Ginsberg M. D., Globus M. Y.-T., Busto R., and Dietrich W. D. (1990) *The Potential Combination Pharmacotherapy in Cerebral Ischemia*. Wissenschaftl Verlagsfesell-schaft, Stuttgart.

5. Shuaib A., Ijaz S., Mazagri R., and Senthilsevlvan A. (1993) CGS-19755 is neuroprotective during repetitive ischemia: this effect is significantly enhanced when combined with hypothermia. *Neuroscience* **56,** 915–920.

6. Guan J., Gunn A. J., Sirimanne E. S., et al. (2000) The window of opportunity for neuronal rescue with insulin-like growth factor-1 after hypoxia-ischemia in rats is critically modulated by cerebral temperature during recovery. *J. Cereb. Blood Flow Metab.* **20,** 513–519.

7. Schmid-Elsaesser R., Hungerhuber E., Zausinger S., Baethmann A., and Reulen H. J. (1999) Combination drug therapy and mild hypothermia: a promising treatment strategy for reversible, focal cerebral ischemia. *Stroke* **30,** 1891–1899.

8. Ogilvy C. S., Chu D., and Kaplan S. (1996) Mild hypothermia, hypertension, and mannitol are protective against infarction during experimental intracranial temporary vessel occlusion. *Neurosurgery* **38,** 1202–1209; discussion 1209–1210.

9. Pazos A. J., Green E. J., Busto R., et al. (1999) Effects of combined postischemic hypothermia and delayed *N*-tert-butyl-alpha-pheylnitrone (PBN) administration on histopathological and behavioral deficits associated with transient global ischemia in rats. *Brain Res.* **846,** 186–195.

10. Westermaier T., Zausinger S., Baethmann A., Steiger H. J., and Schmid-Elsaesser R. (2000) No additional neuroprotection provided by barbiturate-induced burst suppression under mild hypothermic conditions in rats subjected to reversible focal ischemia. *J. Neurosurg.* **93,** 835–844.

11. Meden P., Overgaard K., Pedersen H., and Boysen G. (1994) Effect of hypothermia and delayed thrombolysis in a rat embolic stroke model. *Acta Neurol. Scand.* **90,** 91–98.

12. Wang C. X., Yang T. and Shuaib A. (2003) Effects of minocycline alone and in combination with mild hypothermia in embolic stroke. *Brain Res.* **963,** 327–329.

13. Kahveci F. S., Kahveci N., Alkan T., Goren B., Korfali E., and Ozluk K. (2001) Propofol versus isoflurane anesthesia under hypothermic conditions: effects on intracranial pressure and local cerebral blood flow after diffuse traumatic brain injury in the rat. *Surg. Neurol.* **56,** 206–214.

14. Zausinger S., Westermaier T., Baethmann A., Steiger H. J., and Schmid-Elsaesser R. (2001) Neuroprotective treatment paradigms in neurovascular surgery—efficacy in a rat model of focal cerebral ischemia. *Acta Neurochir. Suppl.* **77,** 259–265.

7

Intraoperative and Intensive Care Management of the Patient Undergoing Mild Hypothermia

Teresa E. Bell-Stephens, RN,
Richard A. Jaffe, MD, PhD,
and Gary K. Steinberg, MD, PhD

INTRODUCTION

Deep hypothermia (18–25°C) as a means of offering neuroprotection has long been accepted and utilized in the operative setting *(1,2)*. It minimizes neuronal injury and death when used in conjunction with cardiopulmonary bypass for cardiac surgery or during craniotomies requiring circulatory arrest and a bloodless field. It is a very effective method of obtaining neuroprotection, but carries some risks, including cardiac arrhythmias, clotting defects, electrolyte abnormalities, and increased rates of infection *(3)*. In addition, deep hypothermia significantly decreases drug metabolism and excretion *(4)*.

Mild hypothermia (33–35°C) is an alternative approach to cerebral protection that is becoming increasingly popular in various clinical settings. Experimental animal studies have shown that temperature reductions of just a few degrees can offer significant neuroprotection following stroke or acute head injury. Although mild hypothermia has far fewer risks when compared with deep hypothermia, it still presents clinical challenges in controlling various physiologic parameters and managing potential complications.

BACKGROUND

Hypothermia has been utilized in several clinical settings since Temple Fay reported its use in an attempt to halt metastatic disease and

From: *Hypothermia and Cerebral Ischemia: Mechanisms and Clinical Applications*
Edited by: C. M. Maier and G. K. Steinberg © Humana Press Inc., Totowa, NJ

offer pain control *(5)*. Patients were placed in tubs of ice water in air-conditioned rooms after being anesthetized. Their core body temperatures were allowed to drift down to as low as 23.3°C for up to 8 d. In some cases, no detectable blood pressure or pulses were present, yet when their body temperatures were normalized, many awakened without neurologic deficits. He reported good pain control for up to a few months with few complications. While his study was novel, his research was not rigorous and no useful data could be gathered from his work. Talbott reported that newly diagnosed schizophrenic patients treated with hypothermia had an improvement in their symptoms for up to 6 mo *(6)*. The enthusiasm for using hypothermia fell out of favor after this for reasons that are unclear, but may have been related to the use of alternative methods of neuroprotection such as barbiturates, which were thought to be more effective.

Several neurosurgeons reported experience with hypothermia in the 1950s, including Botterell, who used moderate hypothermia (28.6–30°C) as a means of neuroprotection during temporary arterial occlusion *(2)*. Overall results were good, but there were several reports of complications, including ventricular arrhythmias and bleeding. Utilization of cardiopulmonary bypass (CPB) with deep hypothermia to achieve a bloodless field in the treatment of giant aneurysms or highly vascular brain tumors was first reported in 1964. Drake et al. described 10 patients undergoing clipping of giant aneurysms using this procedure *(7)*. Outcomes were poor, but this could be attributed to the complexity of the aneurysms, as well as the developmental status of the CPB technique. Utilization of this procedure declined because of the high risk for cardiac complications as well as coagulopathy. By the 1980s, anesthesia was safer and CPB techniques had improved with the use of membrane oxygenators. Silverberg et al. subsequently reported good results using CPB with deep hypothermia in a series of patients with giant aneurysms or vascular tumors *(1)*. Spetzler et al. reported a series of posterior circulation aneurysm clippings done with circulatory arrest, hypothermia, and barbiturates *(8)*. These studies supported earlier reports of effective neuroprotection with deep hypothermia in high-risk surgical cases. Still, the technique was invasive, and patients were at increased risk for bleeding, cardiac arrhythmias, stroke, infection, and other complications.

Mild hypothermia has gained attention in recent years after laboratory studies showed a significant reduction in ischemic neuronal death with just a slight reduction in temperature *(9–13)*. The mechanism of mild hypothermic neuroprotection is not completely understood, but is very likely a result of slowing the progression of the ischemic cascade and pathologic neuroexcitation that is characteristic of all types of brain insult *(10,11,13–16)*. Mild hypothermia reduces the release of glutamate and dopamine into the brain's extracellular spaces. It also attenuates the release of calcium and reduces production of reactive oxygen species *(17,18)*. Lowering the body temperature 3–5°C reduces the anaerobic metabolism and high-energy phosphate depletion *(19–21)*. In addition, mild hypothermia appears to facilitate the resynthesis of ubiquitin following ischemia, promotes postischemic metabolic recovery, decreases neutrophil infiltration and other aspects of inflammation, increases Bcl-2 protein expression, attenuates cytochrome *c* release, and blocks apoptotic neuronal death *(9–11,22–26)*.

Clinical experience using mild hypothermia has been reported in surgical patients as well as in head injury, stroke, and following cardiac arrest. In a feasibility trial, Baker et al. showed that mild hypothermia could be used safely in the operative setting with no untoward effect *(27)*. Specifically, there were no cardiac arrhythmias reported in this series. Steinberg et al. reported a large series of patients undergoing craniotomy for aneurysm clipping or tumor or vascular malformation resection *(28)*. In this series of 459 patients, the complication rate was extremely low. Bleeding was reported in one case of a 32-yr-old male undergoing partial resection of a large (5 cm) Spetzler grade II AVM. He developed disseminated intravascular coagulopathy (DIC) after the bladder temperature reached 32.3°C and the nasoesophageal temperature reached 30.5°C. His initial clinical outcome was poor. However, he made an excellent recovery at a 2-yr follow-up. Another patient undergoing clipping of a middle cerebral and posterior communicating artery aneurysm developed malignant hyperthermia, which was not initially detected until the anesthesiologist noted an elevated end-expired CO2, requiring increased minute ventilation. The typical hyperthermic response was masked because of the use of mild hypothermia. The patient was promptly treated with dantrolene and had no clinical complications. One patient undergoing craniotomy for clipping of internal carotid and posterior communicating artery aneurysms developed monofocal premature ventricular contractions (PVCs) intraoperatively, and had trigeminy during the rewarming phase. There were no alterations in his hemodynamic status and the arrhythmias resolved

Table 1
Stanford Intraoperative Mild Hypothermia Cases
(1991–2003)

Aneurysms	573
Vascular malformations	562
Other craniotomy	424
Total	1559

completely within 24 h postoperatively. To date, we have used intra-operative mild hypothermia in 1559 patients undergoing craniotomy for cerebrovascular procedures or tumor resections (**Table 1**).

Some clinical trials have used mild hypothermia in acute head injury. In a single center study, Clifton et al. reported a series of 46 patients with severe (Glasgow Coma Scores [GCS] 4–7) closed head injury. Patients were randomized to hypothermia vs normothermia within 6 h of injury *(29)*. Hypothermic patient temperatures were kept between 33 and 35°C for 48 h after the target temperature was reached. Normothermic patients were kept at a target temperature of 37°C. Glasgow Outcome Score (GOS) was assessed at 3 mo postinjury by a blinded evaluator. There was no significant improvement in the GOS between the two groups, but a trend toward a better GOS was noted in the hypothermic group. They reported a higher incidence of sepsis in the hypothermic group; however, it was not statistically significant.

Another clinical trial from one institution using mild hypothermia in patients with acute head injury was reported by Marion et al. *(30,31)*. This series showed a significant improvement in the GOS scores of hypothermic patients with initial GCSs between 5 and 7. Mild hypothermia (33°C) was employed for 24 h after the injury. A retrospective review of this series demonstrated no increased incidence of delayed intracerebral hemorrhage in the hypothermic group when compared to the control group *(32)*. Cancio et al. reported a case of a head-injured patient treated with hypothermia induced via peritoneal dialysis (PD) *(33)*. This patient did not have a good neurological outcome on discharge from the hospital. However, hypothermia was achieved using PD without any complications.

A large multicenter trial using mild hypothermia in severe head injury was recently halted as a result of an interim analysis showing the probability of a positive outcome was unlikely *(34)*. However, the study did indicate a potential benefit in patients < 45 yr of age if treatment was begun soon after injury *(35)*. Outcome results were based on GOS at 6 mo. The investigators recommended that further trials are necessary with more stringent uniformity in the management of hemodynamics. They further suggested including only centers where patients are routinely randomized to clinical trials and continuous monitoring of protocol compliance at all participating centers *(36)*.

Recently, several studies have suggested or demonstrated that mild hypothermia may be neuroprotective in patients with acute intracranial hemorrhage or ischemic infarction. Hindman et al. reported a pilot trial using mild hypothermia intraoperatively in 114 patients undergoing aneurysm clipping *(37)*. Patients were randomized to hypothermia (target temperature 33.5°C) or normothermia (target temperature 36.5°C). Neurological evaluations including the National Institutes of Health Stroke Scale (NIHSS), GOS, as well as evaluation of postoperative critical care requirements including respiratory and cardiovascular complications were studied. The results showed a nonsignificant trend in decreased neurological deterioration postoperatively, a greater frequency of discharge to home, and a higher incidence of good long-term outcomes in patients with subarachnoid hemorrhage and ruptured aneurysms randomized to the hypothermic group. A larger multicenter trial is currently underway with no results yet reported.

Schwab et al. used mild hypothermia (33–34°C) in 20 patients with acute severe middle cerebral artery (MCA) infarction for 48–72 h and found mild hypothermia to be safe and feasible *(38)*. Schwab subsequently reported a series of 25 patients with severe MCA infarction treated with the same protocol *(39)*. Intracranial pressure (ICP) was monitored for 3–7 d, and was found to decrease with initiation of hypothermia. ICP increased during rewarming in several patients, but not to the levels seen prior to induction of hypothermia. Pneumonia was seen in 40% of patients treated with hypothermia in this trial, which is within the expected range of occurrence in patients with prolonged ventilation *(40)*. Shimizu et al. used mild hypothermia (33°C) in five patients with embolic infarctions involving the internal carotid artery and MCA territories. The hypothermia was maintained for 3–7 d *(41)*. It was found to be safe, but the number of patients was too small to report any efficacy. Another acute stroke trial using convection air to induce mild hypothermia without anesthesia was found to be feasible *(42)*. Temperatures in this trial were reduced only to 35.5°C, and shivering was controlled with Pethidine. No efficacy was established because of the small number of patients.

Improved neurologic outcomes using mild hypothermia following cardiac arrest was recently reported in two landmark prospective, randomized, controlled studies. In the first study, 275 patients with cardiac arrest from ventricular fibrillation were randomized to mild hypothermia (32–34°C) or normothermia. Target hypothermia temperatures in the treatment group were attained with a mean time of 8 h (range 4–16 h) and were maintained for 24 h. A blinded evaluator assessed the patients at 6 mo using the Pittsburgh cerebral performance scale. Patients randomized to hypothermia ($n = 138$) had lower mortality rates and had significantly improved outcomes compared with the control group *(43)*. Another study of 77 patients with witnessed cardiac arrest from ventricular fibrillation was recently reported. Patients were randomized to mild hypothermia ($n = 43$) vs normothermia ($n = 34$). Hypothermia was initiated outside of the hospital, and the target temperature of 33°C was reached within 2 h of resuscitation and maintained for 12 h in the hypothermia group. A rehabilitation specialist who was blinded to treatment randomization categorized patients as good outcome if they were discharged to home or to a rehabilitation center, and poor outcome if they were discharged to an extended care facility or died. The hypothermia group had a significantly higher rate of good outcomes (55% vs 39% in normothermia) using these criteria *(44)*.

These are the first clinical trials to demonstrate improved outcomes using hypothermia in this population of cardiac arrest patients. However, it's possible that some of the beneficial outcome in these studies was related to the prevention of hyperthermia. Experimental data have shown that even mild hyperthermia contributes to ischemic injury.

POTENTIAL COMPLICATIONS/RISKS
OF MILD HYPOTHERMIA

Mild hypothermia has been easily incorporated into the overall care of patients in various clinical settings. However, there is a potential for multisystem complications when it is used. Although mild hypothermia (32–34°C) is not usually responsible for cardiac dysrhythmias, it has been associated with electrical conduction disturbances secondary to its potentiation of other drugs, particularly neuromuscular blocking agents *(4,45,46)*. There is a tendency to develop atrial fibrillation at temperatures below 32°C *(47)*. During periods of mild hypothermia, there is a shift of potassium to the intracellular space, which increases the potential for arrhythmias. However, replacement of potassium must be done cautiously, as hyperkalemia may occur during rewarming *(48)*.

Coagulation defects have been noted with severe hypothermia. These defects include platelet dysfunction, increased fibrinolytic activity, and decreased enzymatic activity necessary for clotting to occur *(48,49)*. However, even mild surface cooling may produce a reversible platelet defect *(48,50,51)*. Mild hypothermia typically reduces metabolism and hepatic clearance of various anesthetic agents and other medications *(52)*. This must be taken into consideration when formulating an anesthetic plan for the hypothermic patient.

The rate of infection may be higher in patients treated with mild hypothermia. Cutaneous vasoconstriction, which leads to lowered tissue oxygenation subcutaneously, can reduce resistance to infection. In addition, immune function impairment, including neutrophil activity, may be the result of peripheral vasoconstriction and consequent tissue hypoxia *(43,49,50)*.

PATIENT SELECTION FOR TREATMENT WITH MILD HYPOTHERMIA

Patients must be carefully screened and selected for treatment. Because hypothermia may potentiate bleeding disorders, coagulopathic patients should be excluded from this treatment. Routine coagulation studies are done before the body temperature is lowered. Patients with cryoglobulinopathies are also excluded, as hypothermia increases the risk for sickling of the cells. Mild hypothermia should be used cautiously in patients at high risk for infection.

Any history of recent myocardial infarction or arrhythmias should exclude a patient from treatment. An ECG should be examined before treatment is initiated. Continuous cardiac monitoring is essential during the cooling, maintenance, and rewarming periods.

Patients with poor skin integrity or overall poor nutrition are at higher risk for skin breakdown during treatment with mild hypothermia. This should be evaluated when considering appropriateness of treatment. A cloth barrier should be placed between the skin and any cooling devices applied directly to the body to prevent skin trauma.

Pediatric patients tend to cool and rewarm much faster as a result of their high surface to volume ratio. Bissonnette reported a series of 84 pediatric patients weighing between 5 and 50 kg who were observed postoperatively for detrimental effects of mild hypothermia *(53)*. No complications were noted. Specifically, their pulmonary assessment remained stable and there was no prolongation of their postanesthetic recovery. We have used mild intraoperative hypothermia in 80 pediatric craniotomy procedures (ages 6 mo–17 yr) without complications.

METHODS OF COOLING

Hypothermia is easily induced in various clinical settings, and does not require significant allocation of resources. There are various methods of inducing hypothermia. General anesthesia alone is known to lower the core body temperature. Decreasing the room temperature will also assist in this process. Cooling water blankets can be placed underneath and convection air blankets can be placed over patients. Intravenous fluids are often cooled prior to infusion. Ice packs may be placed at skin folds, and gastric and/or bladder lavage with iced solutions may be performed. Fans may be used to circulate cool air for patients in the intensive care unit.

Techniques to improve control of core temperature are currently being studied. One such technique undergoing evaluation at several institutions, including Stanford, is the Innercool Therapies Celsius Control System. This endovascular heat exchanger is inserted into the inferior vena cava (IVC), and cools or rewarms the patient regardless of surface to volume ratio. Saline circulated through the catheter from a console extracts and delivers heat as blood flows around a heat transfer element *(54)*. In our experience using this catheter, patients were generally cooled to 33°C within 30–60 min after cooling was initiated (**Fig. 1**). A recent multicenter randomized clinical trial in 153 patients undergoing elective surgery for unruptured intracranial aneurysms demonstrated cooling rates using the catheter are 4.8°C/h compared with 0.9°C/h in the control group using only forced air surface cooling techniques. Rewarming rates are 1.9°C/h in the catheter group compared to 0.7°C/h in the control group *(55)*. Endovascular cooling in acute ischemic stroke was recently reported in four patients with NIHSS scores between 8 and 25. Patients were cooled to 33°C for 24 h with a heat exchange catheter (SetPoint System, Radiant Medical, Inc.) with mean time to cooling of 7 h 37 min ± 1.7 h. Patients were awake, but sedated with buspirone and meperidine, with a warming blanket to suppress shivering *(56)*. A similar study of endovascular cooling in ischemic stroke patients was

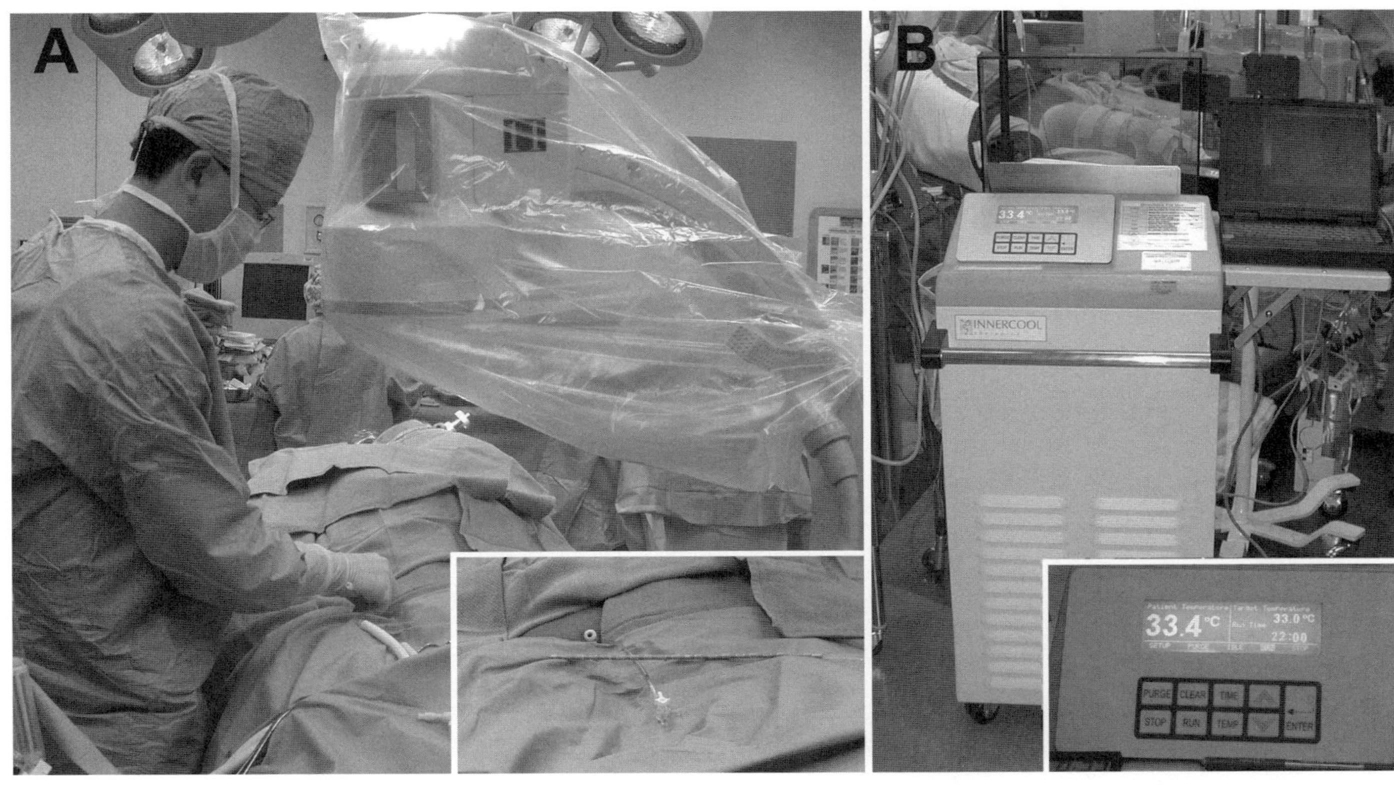

Fig. 1. Patients were cooled to 33°C within 30–60 min using the Innercool Therapies Celsius Control System.

reported in six subjects with MCA infarction using an 8.5-French catheter dwelling in the IVC with cooled normal saline circulating through a close-loop system (ICY®, Alsius Corporation). Patients were cooled to 32.2–33.4°C for 50–78 h (mean 67 ± 13 h). The most common side effects were pneumonia, hypotension, arrhythmia, and thrombocytopenia *(50)*.

Continuous hemodynamic monitoring is essential during all phases of hypothermia. Cardiac monitoring is necessary because of the increased risk of arrhythmias. Cardiac output is decreased 5% for every 1°C of body temperature reduction. This is thought to be secondary to bradycardia, which has been shown to occur with hypothermia *(3)*. A pulmonary artery catheter may be placed if there is any question of hemodynamic instability. Arterial catheters are used for continuous blood pressure measurement, as well as for access to arterial blood for blood gas and electrolyte analysis.

Constant monitoring of body temperature is necessary during the entire process. Core temperature is generally measured via tympanic membrane, rectal, or bladder probes. If esophageal probes are used, they are placed distally, below the tracheal bifurcation. This is to prevent false temperature readings from inspired airway gases. Central venous lines with a temperature probe also allow for core body temperature monitoring. Temperature can be measured via a pulmonary artery catheter when available. Comparisons have been done between brain and body temperature, and good correlation has been shown *(28,31,57)*. If the core temperature falls below the desired level, active rewarming should be initiated.

INTRAOPERATIVE COOLING

Intraoperative hypothermia using surface cooling techniques is started with induction of anesthesia and is continued until approx 0.5°C above the target temperature. Active rewarming should be started and typically results in a further reduction (0.3–0.5°C) in body temperature. This "paradoxical cooling" is the result of surface-heating induced perfusion of cold peripheral tissue, which diverts heat from the core, resulting in further reduction of core temperature. Within 30–60 min, the patient's temperature will have stabilized at or near the target temperature and rewarming is stopped. Subsequent heating and cooling are used as needed to maintain target temperature until the ischemia risk is over (e.g., removal of temporary clips, retractors, etc.). Most patients can be cooled by a combination of surface techniques at the rate of 1°C/30–45 min.

Patients with a low surface to volume ratio may take considerably longer to cool by surface techniques. For these patients additional cooling can be provided by the use of chilled intravenous solutions, bladder irrigation, and gastric lavage.

A long-acting neuromuscular blocking agent (e.g., pancuronium) is administered at the beginning of the case, and rarely requires supplementation. Typically, this minimizes the requirement for anticholinesterases at the end of surgery, which may help reduce the incidence of postoperative nausea and vomiting.

Intraoperative electrophysiologic monitoring is increasingly used during high-risk craniotomies to provide ongoing information about the integrity of motor/sensory pathways as well as cranial nerve function while patients are anesthetized (58,59). General anesthesia is known to cause a decrease in evoked potential amplitudes while increasing component latencies. Mild hypothermia has been found to further reduce somatosensory evoked potential (SSEP) amplitudes (60). Intraoperative electrophysiologic monitoring is used routinely at our institution and a bilateral reduction in the SSEP amplitude is commonly observed. It is therefore important that baseline waveforms be reestablished during the case at each stage of the surgery. The evoked potentials should improve immediately as the patient rewarms and emerges from anesthesia.

Postoperative shivering following mild hypothermia has been associated with increased myocardial oxygen demand, which may lead to myocardial ischemia (48). It can also cause increased intracranial pressure (49). In addition, shivering may result in metabolic acidosis secondary to increased carbon dioxide production. Shivering can be minimized by careful rewarming of the patient before extubation and by using low-dose meperidine or clonidine.

INTENSIVE CARE UNIT CARE

Hypothermia in stroke and head-injured patients is started as soon as possible after injury, and continues for the duration selected by the investigator. Each patient undergoing treatment with mild hypothermia should be paralyzed and sedated to prevent discomfort and reduce shivering. Unfortunately, this can compromise accurate evaluation of the neurological status in patients with acute head injury or stroke. Therefore, continuous monitoring of ICP is important in these intensive care unit patients. Because these patients are paralyzed and sedated, continuous mechanical ventilation is also necessary. Neuromuscular blocking agents are titrated to maintain a single twitch with neuromuscular monitoring to provide for easy reversal of the motor block. Hourly pupil checks should be performed, as well as a daily computerized tomography scan of head. Larson et al. demonstrated that mild hypothermia does not affect the pupil reactivity to light *(61)*. Therefore, any pupil changes should not be assumed to be related to the lowered body temperature.

REWARMING

Rewarming is usually started when the risk of cerebral ischemia has passed. Active rewarming is used in surgical patients. This is accomplished by using a warm air blanket (e.g., Bair Hugger®) in conjunction with water-circulating warm pad and by increasing the operating room temperature. Warming and humidifying inspired gasses, and bladder irrigation with warm saline, may also be used to increase the rate of rewarming. Surgery patients can be rewarmed to 37°C within approx 2–3 h using currently available techniques and within 1–2 h utilizing an intravenous catheter based temperature control system *(55)*.

In protocols for stroke or head injury, normalizing the room temperature and halting all methods of hypothermia accomplished passive rewarming. Normothermia under these conditions is typically accomplished over 12–16 h *(31,34,39)*.

SUMMARY

Mild hypothermia is a practical and safe method for neuroprotection when used properly. Attention to the patient's past medical history, as well as a thorough physical examination is essential prior to instituting hypothermia. It is a relatively inexpensive method that requires minimal resources outside of those that are already standard practice, especially in surgical patients.

Deliberate mild hypothermia has been shown to be an extremely effective means of neuroprotection during periods of ischemia in experimental models. Intraoperative mild hypothermia has become a standard of practice for many neurosurgeons performing complex intracranial procedures. Recent findings of neurologic benefit in prospective, randomized, controlled clinical studies of cardiac arrest patients are encouraging, but more research is required to confirm and extend these positive results to other patients with stroke and traumatic insults. Further investigation must be completed to establish the optimal time and duration when treatment should be instituted to offer the optimal protection for patients with acute ischemic and traumatic injuries.

REFERENCES

1. Silverberg G. D., Reitz B. A., and Ream A. K. (1981) Hypothermia and cardiac arrest in the treatment of giant aneurysms of the cerebral circulation and hemangioblastoma of the medulla. *J. Neurosurg.* **55,** 337–346.
2. Botterell E. H., Lougheed W. M., Morley T. P., and Vaderwater S. L. (1958) Hypothermia in surgical treatment of ruptured intracranial aneurysms. *J. Neurosurg.* **15,** 4–18.
3. Bernard S. (1996) Induced hypothermia in intensive care medicine. *Anaesth. Intens. Care* **24,** 382–388.
4. Heier T., Caldwell J. E., Sessler D. I., and Miller, R. D. (1991) Mild intraoperative hypothermia increases duration of action and recovery time of vecuronium blockade during nitrous oxide-isoflurane anesthesia in humans. *Anesthesiology* **74,** 815–819.
5. Fay T. (1940) Observations on prolonged human refrigeration. *NY State J. Med.* **40,** 1351–1354.
6. Talbott J. H. (1941) The physiologic and therapeutic effects of hypothermia. *N. Engl. J. Med.* **224,** 281–288.
7. Drake C. G., Barr H. W. K., Coles J. G., and Gergely N. F. (1964) The use of extracorporeal circulation and profound hypothermia in the treatment of ruptured intracranial aneurysm. *J. Neurosurg.* **21,** 575–581.
8. Spetzler R. F., Hadley M. N., Rigamonti D., et al. (1988) Aneurysms of the basilar artery treated with circulatory arrest, hypothermia, and barbiturate cerebral protection. *J. Neurosurg.* **68,** 868–879.
9. Ginsberg M. D., Sternau L. L., Globus M., Dietrich W. D., and Busto R. (1992) Therapeutic modulation of brain temperature: relevance to ischemic brain injury. *Cerebrovasc. Brain Metab. Rev.* **4,** 189–225.
10. Maier C. M., Ahern K. vB., Cheng M. L., Lee J. E., Yenari M. A., and Steinberg G. K. (1998) Optimal depth and duration of mild hypothermia in a focal model of transient cerebral ischemia: effects on neurologic outcome, infarct size, apoptosis and inflammation. *Stroke* **29,** 2171–2180.
11. Maier C. M., Sun G. H., Kunis D., Yenari M. A., and Steinberg G. K. (2001) Delayed induction and long-term effects of mild hypothermia in a focal model of transient cerebral ischemia: neurological outcome and infarct size. *J. Neurosurg.* **94,** 90–96.
12. Lo E. H. and Steinberg G. K. (1992) Effects of hypothermia on evoked potentials, magnetic resonance imaging and blood flow in focal cerebral ischemia in rabbits. *Stroke* **23,** 889–893.
13. Lo E. H., Steinberg G. K., Panahian N., Maidment N. T., and Newcomb R. (1993) Profiles of extracellular amino acid changes in focal cerebral ischemia: effects of mild hypothermia. *Neurol. Res.* **15,** 281–287.
14. Busto R., Globus M. Y-T, Dietrich W. D., Martinez E., Valdes I., and Ginsberg M. D. (1998b) Effect of mild hypothermia on ischemia-induced release of neurotransmitters and free fatty acids in rat brain. *Stroke* **20,** 904–910.
15. Baker A. J., Fiore A. J., Franzzini V. I., Choudhri T. F., Zubay G. P., and Solomon R. A. (1995) Intraischemic hypothermia decreases the release of glutamate in the cores of permanent focal cerebral infarcts. *Neurosurgery* **36,** 994–1001.
16. Nakashima K. and Todd M. M. (1996) Effects of hypothermia, pentobarbital and Isoflurane on postdepolarization amino acid release during global cerebral ischemia. *Anesthesiology* **85,** 161–168.

17. Maier C. M., Yenari M. A., Chan P. H., and Steinberg G. K. (2000) Effects of mild hypothermia on superoxide production following transient focal cerebral ischemia. *Stroke* **31,** 339.

18. Maier C. M., Sun G. H., Cheng D., Yenari M. A., Chan P. H., and Steinberg G. K. (2002) Effects of mild hypothermia on superoxide anion production and superoxide dismutase expression following transient focal cerebral ischemia. *Neurobiol. Dis.* **11,** 28–42.

19. Rosomoff H. L. and Holaday D. A. (1954) Cerebral blood flow and cerebral oxygen consumption during hypothermia. *Am. J. Physiol.* **4,** 85–88.

20. Croughwell N., Smith L. R., Quill T., et al. (1992) The effect of temperature on cerebral metabolism and blood flow in adults during cardiopulmonary bypass. *J. Thorac. Cardiovasc. Surg.* **103,** 549–554.

21. Colbourne F., Sutherland G., and Corbett D. (1997) Postischemic hypothermia. A critical appraisal with implications for clinical treatment. *Mol. Neurobiol.* **14,** 171–201.

22. Zhang Z. J., Sobel R. A., Cheng D., Steinberg G. K., and Yenari M. A. (2001) Mild hypothermia increases Bcl-2 protein expression following global cerebral ischemia. *Mol. Brain Res.* **95,** 75–85.

23. Yenari M. A., Iwayama S., Cheng D., et al. (2002) Mild hypothermia attenuates cytochrome c release but does not alter Bcl-2 expression or caspase activation after experimental stroke. *J. Cereb. Blood Flow Metab.* **22,** 29–38.

24. Xu L., Yenari M. A., Steinberg G. K., and Giffard R. (2002) Mild hypothermia reduces apoptosis of mouse neurons *in vitro* early in the cascade. *J. Cereb. Blood Flow Metab.* **22,** 21–28.

25. Soo H. H., Qiao Y., Karabiyikoglu M., Giffard R. G., and Yenari M. A. (2002) Influence of mild hypothermia on inducible nitric oxide synthase expression and reactive nitrogen production in experimental stroke and inflammation. *J. Neurosci.* **22,** 3921–3928.

26. Yamashita K., Eguchi Y., Kajiwara K., and Ito H. (1991) Mild hypothermia ameliorates ubiquitin synthesis and prevents delayed neuronal death in gerbil hippocampus. *Stroke* **22,** 1574–1581.

27. Baker K. Z., Young W. L., Stone J. G., Kader A., Baker C. J., and Solomon R. A. (1994) Deliberate mild intraoperative hypothermia for craniotomy. *Anesthesiology* **81,** 361–367.

28. Steinberg G. K., Grant G., and Yoon E. (1995) Deliberate hypothermia. In *Intraoperative Neuroprotection* (Andrews R. J., ed.), Williams & Wilkins, Baltimore, pp. 65–85.

29. Clifton G. L., Allen S., Barrodale P., et al. (1993) A phase II study of moderate hypothermia in severe brain injury. *J. Neurotrauma* **10,** 263–271.

30. Marion D. W., Obrist W. D., Carlier P. M., Penrod L. E., and Darby J. M. (1993) The use of moderate therapeutic hypothermia for patients with severe head injuries: a preliminary report. *J. Neurosurg.* **79,** 354–362.

31. Marion D. W., Penrod L. E., Kelsey S. F., et al. (1997) Treatment of traumatic brain injury with moderate hypothermia. *N. Engl. J. Med.* **336,** 540–546.

32. Resnick D. K., Marion D. W., and Darby J. M. (1994) The effect of hypothermia on the incidence of delayed traumatic intracerebral hemorrhage. *Neurosurgery* **34,** 252–256.

33. Cancio L. C., Wortham W. G., and Zimba F. (1994) Peritoneal dialysis to induce hypothermia in a head injured patient: case report. *Surg. Neurol.* **42,** 303–307.

34. Clifton G. L., Miller E. R., Choi S. C., et al. (2001) Lack of effect of induction of hypothermia after acute brain injury. *N. Engl. J. Med.* **344,** 556–563.

35. Clifton G. L. (2000) Hypothermia in acute brain injury. *Neurosci. Res. Center News* **7,** 1–2.

36. Clifton G. L., Sung C. C., Miller E. R., et al. (2001) Intercenter variance in clinical trials of head trauma-experience of the National Acute Brain Injury Study: Hypothermia. *J. Neurosurg.* **95,** 751–755.

37. Hindman B. J., Todd M. M., Gelb A. W., et al. (1999) Mild hypothermia as a protective therapy during intracranial aneurysm surgery: a randomized prospective pilot trial. *Neurosurgery* **44,** 23–32.

38. Schwab S., Schwartz M., Aschoff A., Keller E., and Hacke W. (1998) Moderate hypothermia and brain temperature in patients with severe middle cerebral artery infarction. *Acta Neurochir. Suppl.* **71,** 131–134.

39. Schwab S., Schwarz S., Spranger M., Keller E., Bertram M., and Hacke W. (1998) Moderate hypothermia in the treatment of patients with severe middle cerebral artery infarction. *Stroke* **29,** 2461–2466.

40. Chevret S., Hemmer M., Carlet J., and Langer M. (1993) Incidence and risk factors of pneumonia acquired in intensive care units: results from a multicenter prospective study on 996 patients. *Intens. Care Med.* **19,** 256–264.

41. Shimizu T., Naritomi H., Oe H., et al. (1996) Mild hypothermia prevents the development of cerebral edema and hemorrhagic transformation in acute embolic stroke. *Cerebrovasc. Dis.* **(Suppl 2),** 32–178.

42. Kammersgaard L. P., Rasmussen B. H., Jorgensen H. S., Reith J., Weber U., and Olsen T. S. (2000) Feasibility and safety of inducing modest hypothermia in awake patients with acute stroke through surface cooling: a case-control study. *Stroke* **31,** 2251–2256.

43. The Hypothermia After Cardiac Arrest Study Group. (2002) Mild therapeutic hypothermia to improve the neurologic outcome after cardiac arrest. *N. Engl. J. Med.* **346,** 549–556.

44. Bernard S. A., Gray T. W., Buist M. D., et al. (2002) Treatment of comatose survivors of out of hospital cardiac arrest with induced hypothermia. *N. Engl. J. Med.* **346,** 557–563.

45. Ham J., Stanski D. R., and Newfield P. (1981) Pharmacokinetics and dynamics of d-tubocurarine during hypothermia in humans. *Anesthesiology* **55,** 631–635.

46. Freysz M., Timour Q., Mazze R. I., et al. (1989) Potentiation by mild hypothermia of ventricular conduction disturbances and reentrant arrhythmias induced by bupivacaine in dogs. *Anesthesiology* **70,** 799–804.

47. Okada M. (1984) The cardiac rhythm in accidental hypothermia. *J. Electrocardiol.* **17,** 123–128.

48. Schubert A. (1992) Should mild hypothermia be routinely used for human cerebral protection? The flip side. *J. Neurosurg. Anesthesiol.* **4(3),** 216–220.

49. Sessler D. I. (1995) Deliberate mild hypothermia. *J. Neurosurg. Anesthesiol.* **7,** 38–46.

50. Georgiadis D., Schwarz S., Kollmar R., and Schwab S. (2001) Endovascular cooling for moderate hypothermia in patients with acute ischemic stroke. *Stroke* **32,** 2550–2553.

51. Valeri C., Feingold H., Cassidy G., Ragno G., Khuri S., and Altschule M. D. (1987) Hypothermia-induced reversible platelet dysfunction. *Ann. Surg.* **205,** 175–181.

52. Leslie K., Sessler D. I., Bjorksten A. R., and Moayeri A. (1995) Mild hypothermia alters propofol pharmacokinetics and increases the duration of action of atracurium. *Anesth. Analg.* **80,** 1007–1014.
53. Bissonnette B. and Sessler D. I. (1993) Mild hypothermia does not impair postanesthetic recovery in infants and children. *Anesth. Analg.* **76,** 168–172.
54. Inderbitzen B., Yon S., Lasheras J., Dobak J., Perl J., and Steinberg G. K. (2002) Safety and performance of a novel intravascular catheter for induction and reversal of hypothermia in a porcine model. *Neurosurgery* **50,** 364–370.
55. Steinberg G. K., Bell-Stephens T. E., Shuer L. M., et al. (2003) Comparison of endovascular cooling to surface-cooling during unruptured cerebral aneurysm repair. *Stroke* **34,** 246.
56. DeGeorgia M. A., Abou-Chebl A., Krieger D. W., Andrefsky J. C., Sila C. A., and Furlan A. J. (2002) Endovascular cooling for patients with acute ischemic stroke. *Stroke* **33,** 271.
57. Mellergard P. and Nordstrom C. (1991) Intracerebral temperature in neurosurgical patients. *Neurosurgery* **28,** 709–713.
58. Lopez J. R., Chang S. D., and Steinberg G. K. (1999) The utility of electrophysiological monitoring during microsurgery of cerebral aneurysms. *J. Neurol. Neurosur. Ps.* **66,** 189–196.
59. Chang S. D., Lopez J. R., and Steinberg G. K. (1999) The usefulness of electrophysiological monitoring during resection of central nervous system vascular malformations. *J. Stroke Cerebrovasc. Dis.* **8,** 412–422.
60. Kochs E. (1995) Electrophysiological monitoring and mild hypothermia. *J. Neurosurg. Anesth.* **7,** 222–228.
61. Larson M. D., Sessler D. I., McGuire J., and Hynson J. M. (1991) Isoflurane, but not mild hypothermia, depresses the human pupillary light reflex. *Anesthesiology* **75,** 62–67.

8

Management of Traumatic Brain Injury With Moderate Hypothermia

Elad I. Levy, MD,
and Donald W. Marion, MD

OVERVIEW

Early reports of therapeutic hypothermia for severe traumatic brain injury can be traced back to the first half of the 20th century. It is only within the last two decades that clinical studies have demonstrated that therapeutic moderate hypothermia for brief durations can improve patient outcomes following brain injury. The historical background, recent clinical experience, and mechanisms of action of moderate hypothermia are reviewed.

EARLY EXPERIENCE

As early as 1943, clinicians began reporting on the use of hypothermia to treat patients with severe traumatic brain injury *(1)*. In this early report, surface cooling techniques were used to cool patients, as low as 24°C. Some patients were kept at these hypothermic temperatures for periods as long as 5 d. This early study demonstrated mixed results in that hypothermia may have contributed to the death of 19 patients, but improvement in the neurologic status of some patients was observed following a 3–4 degree reduction in body temperature. Other reports with similar findings rapidly emerged *(2–5)*. Another investigator used temperatures as low as 28°C to treat 30 patients with hypothermia for 58 h to 6 wk, either continually or intermittently. He found that body temperatures consistently below 30°C resulted in potentially life-threatening infection and cardiac arrhythmias *(4)*. By 1962, Drake, Hendrick,

From: *Hypothermia and Cerebral Ischemia: Mechanisms and Clinical Applications*
Edited by: C. M. Maier and G. K. Steinberg © Humana Press Inc., Totowa, NJ

Lazorthes, and Sedzimir all reported on the use of therapeutic hypothermia for traumatic brain injury (TBI) *(2–4,6)*. Their combined experience involved 115 patients managed at temperatures ranging from 28 to 34°C. Mortality rates were as high as 72%, and approximately one third of these deaths occurred during the rewarming phase. Despite these high mortality rates, each investigator believed that hypothermia had clinical utility and warranted further exploration. In 1974, Shapiro's group reported their experience with barbiturate-augmented moderate hypothermia for patients with TBI *(7)*. He noted that sustained reductions in intracranial pressure (ICP) and improvements in cerebral perfusion pressure (CPP) could be maintained for 5 d using a combination of hypothermia and pentobarbital.

None of these early studies, however, prospectively compared the outcomes of hypothermia-treated patients with those kept at normal temperatures. Comparisons among the different studies were difficult, as depth and duration of cooling and time from injury to initiation of hypothermia varied greatly, both within and among the studies. Many of the patients were cooled below 28°C, resulting in an increase in cardiac arrhythmias and coagulation disorders *(8,9)*. By the late 1960s, surface cooling techniques to achieve profound hypothermia were no longer used because of an increased rate of cardiac arrhythmias, most commonly ventricular fibrillation, which occurred at temperatures below 27°C *(10,11)*. During the past decade, however, several investigators demonstrated that deep hypothermia (<30°C) may not be necessary to provide a significant improvement in functional outcome following experimental brain injury. Studies using ischemia, fluid-percussion, and controlled cortical contusion animal models have demonstrated significant histologic preservation and behavioral improvement with postinjury cooling to 30–33°C for 1–4 h *(12–16)*. This level of cooling has not been shown to cause an increase in cardiac arrhythmias, coagulation disorders, or other medical problems often observed in patients cooled below 27°C *(17–20)* as compared with normothermic traumatic brain-injured patients.

CONTEMPORARY CLINICAL STUDIES

During the last 10 yr the results of five trials of therapeutic mild to moderate hypothermia for the treatment of severe TBI have been published (**Table 1**) *(17,20–23)*. Although there were slight differences in the duration of cooling (1 vs 2 d) and time to initiation of cooling (within

Table 1
Hypothermia Trials: Patient Characteristics and Clinical Outcomes

Study	Randomized	Target temperature	No. of patients in study	Mean age (yr)	Mean GCS	Time to initiate cooling	Good outcome (GOS 4–5): hypothermia group (f/u)	Good outcome (GOS 4–5): normothermia group (f/u)
Jiang et al. (23)	Yes	33–35°C	43	41	5.1	Immediately	47%	27%
Metz et al. (21)	No	32.5–33°C	10	31	3.5	16 h	70% (6 mo)	N/A
Shiozaki et al. (20)	Yes	33.5–34.5°C	33	35	5.2	After failed routine ICP therapy	38% (6 mo)	6% (6 mo)
Clifton et al. (17)	Yes	32–33°C	46	29	5.6	6 h	50% (3 mo)	36% (3 mo)
Marion et al. (22)	Yes	32–33°C	82	33	4.7	6 h	55%[a] (6 mo)	33% (3 mo)
							73%[b] (6 mo)	35% (6 mo)

[a]Percentage of all patients in the study. Differences statistically significant at $p < 0.05$.
[b]Percentage of patients with initial GCS scores of 5–7. Differences statistically significant at $p < 0.01$.

121

hours after injury vs after failure of all other conventional means to control ICP), all patients in the hypothermia groups of these studies showed a trend toward improved clinical outcomes. Other prospective randomized studies demonstrated statistically significant clinical outcomes following management with moderate hypothermia *(22,23)*.

The study by Clifton et al. involved 46 consecutive patients in which the treatment group was cooled to 32–33°C for 48 h. Cooling was initiated within 6 h of injury *(17)*. Patients were rewarmed over 16 h. Glasgow Outcome Scores (GOS) were combined into two categories for analysis: Good Recovery/Moderate Disability (GR/MD) and Severe Disability/Vegetative State/Death (SD/VS/D). At 3 mo after injury 52% of the hypothermia patients were in the GR/MD group and 47% were in the SD/VS/D group. Of the hypothermia patients, 36% were in the GR/MD group and 63% were in the SD/VS/D group. Although Clifton failed to demonstrate a significant improved outcome in the hypothermia group, 30% more patients in the hypothermia group did have moderate, mild, or no disabilities as compared to the normothermia group.

Interestingly, this study differed from the other clinical studies in that the hypothermia group did not appear to have a reduction in ICP (**Table 2**). This may be related to the fact that this study used a fiberoptic white matter catheter to measure ICP, whereas the other studies used a ventriculostomy catheter *(24)*. Similar to some earlier studies, there was an increased incidence of sepsis and coagulation disorders in the hypothermia group. The incidence of cardiac arrhythmias and pneumonia, however, was not significantly different between the two groups. The decrease in the incidence of early seizures in the hypothermic group was statistically significant.

Shiozaki et al. *(20)* studied the effect of hypothermia in 33 patients with severe TBI. Hypothermia was used after conventional measures such as hyperventilation, mannitol, and barbiturate therapy failed to control ICP. All patients with ICPs >20 mmHg following 6 h of high-dose barbiturate therapy were randomized to a control group (normal temperature) or a hypothermic group (33.5–34.5°C). The study group, consisting of 16 patients, was managed with hypothermia for 48 h followed by rewarming to 37°C over the next 48 h. At 6 mo follow-up, good outcomes (mild, moderate, or no disability) were achieved by 38% of those in the hypothermia group and only 6% of the normothermia patients (differences not significant). These investigators found that hypothermia patients achieved a significant decrease in other parameters

Table 2
Effects of Hypothermia on Cerebral Metabolism and Blood Flow as Compared to Normothermic Controls

Study	CBF	CMRO$_2$	ICP	CPP	Heart rate
Jiang et al. (23)	?	?	Decreased	No change	No change
Metza et al. (21)	No change	Decreased	Decreased	No change	No change
Shiozaki et al. (20)	Decreased	Decreased	Decreased	Increased	?
Clifton et al. (17)	?	?	No change	Decreased	Decreased
Marion et al. (22)	Decreased	?	Decreased	Increased	Decreased

[a]In this study, each parameter was compared to values prior to cooling of individual patients.
CBF, Cerebral blood flow; CMRO$_2$, cerebral metabolic rate for oxygen; ICP, intracranial pressure; CPP, cerebral perfusion pressure.

such as cerebral metabolic rate of oxygen ($CMRO_2$) and cerebral blood flow (CBF) with an increase in the CPP ($p = 0.01$; **Table 2**). Unlike many of the early clinical studies, this study showed no difference in the incidence of pneumonia, cardiac arrhythmias, or sepsis between the normothermia and hypothermia groups. An important finding in this study was a statistically significant increase in survival in patients randomized to the hypothermia group. Fifty percent of the patients in the hypothermia group survived vs 18% of the control group ($p = 0.05$).

A follow-up study by these authors examined the outcomes of 62 patients treated with moderate hypothermia. In this group of patients, ICP management was attempted with conventional techniques such as fluid restriction, hyperventilation, and barbiturate therapy *(20)*. Only after elevations in ICP persisted following high barbiturate therapy was hypothermia instituted. Mild hypothermia was induced through surface cooling techniques, and was continued for 2 d or until it was believed to be no longer effective. At 6 mo following the initial TBI, 20% had a favorable outcome, but 65% died.

In 1996, Metz et al. *(21)* described their findings after cooling 10 consecutive patients with severe TBI. Patients were cooled to target temperatures or warmed to 37°C. Some significant drawbacks of the study were that the sample size was small ($n = 10$), and the study was not randomized. Despite these limitations, seven of the 10 patients had only mild, moderate, or no disabilities. Of the remaining three patients, one was severely disabled and the other two died. Hypothermia led to a significant decrease in the ICP with $CMRO_2$ reduced by 45% in these patients ($p = 0.01$). CBF, however, did not change significantly. Prior to initiation of treatment with moderate hypothermia, 6 of the 10 patients had elevated cerebral metabolic rates for lactate (CMRL) indicating cerebral ischemia. Cooling normalized CMRL in all patients ($p = 0.01$). Another important finding in this study was that the study group and the control group did not differ significantly in rates of cardiac arrhythmias, coagulation profile disturbances, or potassium levels.

A prospective, single-center randomized study by Marion et al. *(22)* in 1997 studied 82 consecutive patients randomized to a control group or a study group in which cooling began within 6 h of injury. Patients in the study group were cooled to target temperatures of 32–33°C for 24 h, then rewarmed to 37°C over 12 h. An important finding in this study was that only patients with an initial GCS of 5–7 benefited from moderate hypothermia. The improvement in outcomes seen in the hypothermia groups as compared with the normothermia group was significant at 3 ($p = 0.01$), 6 ($p = 0.01$), and at 12 mo ($p = 0.05$) following injury. At 6 mo follow-up from the time of initial injury, only 35% of the normothermia patients with initial Glasgow Coma Score (GCS) of 5–7 had achieved a good outcome, whereas 73% of the hypothermia patients had demonstrated good outcomes. As seen in earlier studies, the hypothermia patients had a significant reduction in ICP ($p = 0.01$). Interestingly, the study by Marion et al. *(22)* demonstrated significant reductions in CBF in patients treated with hypothermia, whereas the study by Metz et al. *(21)* did not.

Cerebrospinal fluid (CSF) levels in interleukin-1β (IL-1β) and glutamate were significantly lower in the hypothermia group compared to the normothermia group of patients with an initial GCS of 5–7 (**Table 3**). No differences in aspartate levels were found.

In the study by Marion et al. *(22)*, the patients randomized to hypothermic management had significantly lower mean ICP ($p = 0.01$), heart rate ($p = 0.001$), and CBF ($p = 0.05$) observed during the first 36 h of treatment. Mean CPP was higher in the cooled patients as compared to normothermic controls ($p = 0.05$) (**Table 4**). Differences in serum concentrations of glucose, amylase, creatinine, prothrombin time (PT), and hematocrit were not significant. There were no significant differences in the incidence of cardiac arrhythmias, pneumonia, sepsis, or abnormal coagulation parameters between the two groups.

Jiang et al. *(23)* reported findings following the use of mild hypothermia therapy (33–35°C) in 87 patients with severe TBI. From 1992 to 1998, 87 patients with severe TBI were randomly entered into the normothermia group ($n = 44$) or the mild hypothermia group ($n = 43$). In this study, patients in the hypothermia groups were immediately cooled with surface cooling blankets. Patients were cooled 3–14 d, and were rewarmed on return of normal ICP measurements at a rate of 1°C per hour. Patient outcomes at one year demonstrated a mortality rate of 25% in the hypothermia group vs 45% in the normothermia group. Favorable outcomes (good recovery or moderate disability) were achieved in 46% of the hypothermia group and 27% of the normothermia group at 1 yr ($p < 0.05$).

Differences in ICP were noted between the hypothermia and normothermia group in this study. On postinjury d 7, the mean ICP in the hypothermia group was almost 10 mmHg lower than that of the normothermia group ($p < 0.1$). At 1 yr following initial injury, there were no

Table 3
The University of Pittsburgh Study: Statistically Significant Differences in Patients With Initial GCS 5-723

	No. of patients	GOS of 4–5 at 3 mo	GOS 4–5 at 6 mo	GOS 4–5 at 12 mo	CSF IL-1β (pg/mL)	CSF glutamate (mg/dL)
Hypothermia	22	12 (54%)	16 (73%)	16 (73%)	3.1 ± 3.5	0.04 ± 0.02
Normothermia	26	5 (19%)	9 (34%)	10 (38%)	21.5 ± 3.9	0.07 ± 0.05
p Value		0.01	0.01	0.01	0.03	<0.001

Data from ref. 22.
CSF, Cerebrospinal fluid.

Table 4
The University of Pittsburgh Study: Intracranial Physiological Differences Following Hypothermia

	Mean ICP (mmHg)	Mean CPP (mmHg)	Cerebral blood flow (ml/100 g of tissue/min)	Heart rate (beats/min)
Hypothermia	15.4	82.4	28.8	67.4
Normothermia	19.7	77.4	35.7	82.1
p Value	0.01	0.05	0.05	<0.001

Data from ref. 22.

significant differences in the two groups when comparing complication rates of seizure, stress ulcer, pneumonia, and cardiac arrhythmias ($p > 0.05$).

A multicenter trial on the use of therapeutic moderate hypothermia for 48 h in patients with severe traumatic brain injury was reported by Clifton et al. *(25)*. Three hundred and ninety-two patients between the ages of 16 and 65 yr, with an admission GCS score of 8 or less, were randomly assigned to a normothermia group, or to a group who were cooled to 33°C for 48 h and then rewarmed over the next 24 h. In every other way, both groups of patients were treated similarly. The primary outcome measure was the GOS, which was assessed at 6 mo after injury by examiners who were blinded to the patients' treatment group assignments. At that time of outcome assignment, 17 of the patients were unavailable. Of the remaining 368 patients, there were no significant differences between neurologic outcomes in the hypothermia and normothermia groups. Approximately 57% of patients in both groups suffered severe disability, vegetative state, or death (poor outcome) and 43% had good outcomes. Hypothermia was observed to reduce significantly the incidence of intracranial hypertension as compared to the normothermia group, and in patients 45 yr of age and younger who were normovolemic, there was a trend toward improved outcomes in the hypothermia group. Failure of hypothermia to cause improved outcomes in the group as a whole could not be attributed to delay in cooling, as patients who did not reach target temperature until 9 h after injury actually had slightly better outcomes than those who reached target temperature within 2–3 h after injury. This in part may be related to the observation of others that hypothermia on admission to the trauma center is independently associated with poor outcomes.

As a result of this important multicenter trial *(25)*, studies are now focusing on the more effective prevention of fever *(26)*. Others are looking at specific subgroups of patients who may benefit from therapeutic moderate hypothermia, such as younger patients *(27)*. Finally, it is possible that subtle intercenter variations in medical management of severely head-injured patients may have influenced the outcomes of the trial by Clifton et al. *(25)*.

It has been reported that increases in temperature may accentuate brain injury and worsen outcome following stroke and severe TBI *(28–30)*. A recent study by Jiang et al. *(31)* looked at a number of factors that may play an important role in predicting outcome in 846 cases of severe TBI. In that study, the authors found that the outcomes were strongly correlated with GCS score, age, pupillary response and size, hypoxia, hyperthermia, and high ICP.

EXPERIMENTAL EVIDENCE SUPPORTING MODERATE HYPOTHERMIA

Over the past decade, animal models have supported the theory that moderate hypothermia improves behavioral outcomes following severe traumatic brain injury *(12,14,15,29,32–34)*. In a rodent model of fluid-percussion injury, Clifton et al. *(35)* demonstrated a linear dose–response relationship between balance beam performance testing and depth of hypothermia following closed head injury. They found that postinjury treatment with moderate hypothermia resulted in greater reductions in performance deficits for 5 d following injury with cooling to 30°C. Well-designed global ischemia models have found significant neuronal protection with both intraischemic and postischemic hypothermia. In 1987, Busto et al. *(36)* demonstrated a reduction in neuronal injury with 3–4°C hypothermia following four-vessel occlusion in rats. In other global-ischemia models, severe neuronal loss was inhibited by 3 h of hypothermia at 30°C initiated 10 min following four-vessel occlusion *(37)*. Other groups demonstrated that hypothermia of 34°C provided neuronal protection superior to pharmacological methods alone *(38)*. In some of the models, the protective effect of moderate hypothermia was demonstrated when hypothermia was used only following brain injury or onset of brain ischemia *(39)*. Several animal models support the benefits of immediate cooling following initial brain injury. One such canine epidural balloon-compression model demonstrated significant reductions in volume of parenchymal damage when cooling was initiated 15 min after injury as compared with normothermic controls *(40)*. Other rodent models have demonstrated similar results (**Table 5**) *(41)*. Postinjury moderate hypothermia (32–34°C), however, has not been consistently shown to be superior to mild hypothermia (34–36°C) with respect to behavioral improvement and neuronal protection *(15)*.

Several animal models suggest that the time to initiate cooling following TBI is brief. Some rat models suggest that the therapeutic window for treatment with hypothermia is approx 25 min *(41,42)*. These data would seem quite discouraging, as most traumatic brain injury patients do not arrive at the hospital and receive complete evaluation until significantly more time has elapsed. Even with rapid transporta-

Table 5
Therapeutic Moderate Hypothermia in Experimental Traumatic Brain Injury Models

Study	Year	Species	Depth of cooling	Duration of cooling	Outcome
Clifton et al. *(35)*	1991	Rat	30–36°C	1 h	Improved behavior
Jiang et al. *(104)*	1992	Rat	30°C	1 h	Improved BBB integrity
Dietrich et al. *(12)*	1994	Rat	30°C	3 h	Improved histologic preservation
Lyeth et al. *(42)*	1993	Rat	30°C	1 h	Improved behavior
Palmer et al. *(92)*	1994	Rat	32–33°C	4 h	Improved histologic preservation
Pomeranz et al. *(40)*	1993	Dog	31°C	5 h	Improved histologic preservation
Taft et al. *(62)*	1993	Rat	30°C	3 h	Increased microtubule protection
Marion and White *(41)*	1996	Rat	32–33°C	4 h	Improved histologic preservation

tion and expedient evaluation, the earliest most patients can have cooling initiated is approx 2 h after the injury.

The clinical studies reviewed above either suggested or demonstrated improved outcomes with hypothermia, even though cooling was not initiated for up to 24 or 48 h after injury. Analysis of these clinical trials reveals that improved outcomes were achieved in studies that attempted to cool patients as soon as possible after injury as well as in those where there was a substantial delay before initiation of cooling. Perhaps the therapeutic window of hypothermic benefit is species specific. It is not possible to determine if there is a benefit to earlier vs later cooling initiation times from analysis of clinical trials owing to significant methodological differences, but animal studies suggest that better outcomes might be expected with the earliest possible initiation of treatment with hypothermia *(43)*.

MECHANISMS OF THE HYPOTHERMIC EFFECT

Following TBI, a secondary brain injury (i.e., evolving injury following the initial insult) results from dysfunction in normal physiologic and metabolic processes. Many biologic processes are modulated by temperature, and hypothermia may thereby control the cascade of multiple pathophysiologic processes known to result from TBI. Evidence supporting the theory of secondary brain injury is provided by the observation that many victims of severe TBI are conscious immediately after injury but then lose consciousness as time elapses *(44)*; histologic and cytochemical evidence suggests that axonal disruption often occurs hours after the initial impact rather than immediately *(45)*; and the finding of elevated CSF levels of neurochemical mediators of secondary injury days after the impact *(46)*. The pathophysiologic processes implicated as the cause of secondary brain injury include ischemia *(47)*, metabolic alterations *(48,49)*, widespread depolarization *(50)*, amino acid excitotoxicity *(51–53)*, and vascular injury with disruption of the blood–brain barrier (BBB) *(54,55)*. In addition to positively affecting these abnormalities, hypothermia has been shown to reduce free fatty acid production *(56)*, cerebral edema *(57,58)*, leukotriene production *(59)*, intracranial pressure *(58)*, free radical reactions *(60)*, abnormal acetylcholine and dopamine levels *(61)*, and the relative loss of microtubule-associated protein that normally follows TBI (**Table 5**) *(62)*.

During the last decade there have been many randomized clinical trials attempting to identify therapies that are effective in improving outcome following severe TBI. Although these studies used a wide range of target temperatures, only those that utilized moderate hypothermia have demonstrated efficacy in both the laboratory and clinical setting. A possible explanation for the success of hypothermia and failure of the other drug trials is that hypothermia modulates multiple mechanisms of secondary brain injury, while most of the pharmacological studies were focused on a single mechanism *(63)*. Some of these mechanisms are discussed in detail below and in Chapter 4.

CEREBRAL METABOLISM AND OXYGEN CONSUMPTION

Immediately after a severe TBI, there is a substantial reduction in CBF combined with an early hypermetabolic state that leads to regional, and in some cases global, ischemia. Significantly reduced CBF has been demonstrated after severe TBI in rodents *(64)*, baboons *(65)*, and in several human studies *(66–68)*. In a rat subdural hematoma model, severe ischemic damage of the hemisphere underlying the hematoma was associated with a 142% increase in the cerebral metabolic rate of glucose *(68–71)*. Hypothermia reduces normal cerebral metabolism and oxygen consumption by about 7% per degree Celsius *(72–74)*. Other studies demonstrate that the rate of glucose utilization decreased by 35–50% when brain temperatures are 5°C in uninjured rats *(75)*. This observation occurred most commonly in the cortical tissue underlying the hematoma. Others have also documented a marked increase in cerebral metabolism during the first few minutes after fluid percussion injury in the rat *(76)*, a phenomenon that is abolished by three different glutamate antagonists *(77)*. The combination of increased metabolism and decreased CBF may result in profound ischemia with irreversible deficits. Early management with hypothermia may prevent such secondary brain injury. In canine studies, hypothermia caused a 7% decrease in CBF and $CMRO_2$ per degree reduction in body temperature between 35 and 25°C *(78,79)*. In an interesting study by Kuluz et al. *(80)*, selective brain cooling to 31°C with body temperature maintained at normal temperatures resulted in significantly increased CBF as measured by laser Doppler flowmetry.

Despite the fact that some clinical TBI studies also have shown significant reductions in CBF and $CMRO_2$ during cooling (**Table 2**) *(18,20)*, it remains unclear whether the global reduction of cerebral metabolism is sufficient to improve clinical outcomes of patients with severe TBI. In several animal models of ischemia, investigators have shown that reducing cerebral activity with inhalation anesthetics does not lead to a significant reduction in the degree of brain tissue injury *(13,81,82)*. However, most studies examining the cerebral effects of anesthetics measured their efficacy in terms of suppression of cerebral electrical activity induced by those anesthetics. It has been hypothesized that anesthetic agents depress only the component of substrate utilization associated with electrophysiological activity *(24,83)*. Interestingly, a recent study by Kahveci et al. *(84)* showed that propofol anesthesia may be better for use in combination with hypothermia in cases of TBI, as it reduces ICP and increases CPP.

Ion Homeostasis

Ischemia has been shown to deplete high-energy phosphate compounds and cause membrane decomposition, thus losing the ability to maintain intracellular/extracellular ionic homeostasis *(85,86)*. Widespread depolarization due to inactivation of membrane-associated energy-dependent enzyme leads to the efflux of potassium, influx of calcium, collapse of the normal intracellular/extracellular sodium gradient, and eventual reversal of excitatory amino acid (EAA) uptake *(53)*. In some ischemia models, increases in free cytosolic calcium are reduced by moderate hypothermia *(87)*. Others have shown a reduction of calcium in hippocampal slices following infusion of a hypothermic medium *(88)*. These reductions in anoxic depolarization causing intracellular calcium influx with concomitant extracellular flow of potassium are thought to mitigate neuronal injury resulting from associated increases in extracellular levels of EAAs (glutamate, aspartate), acetylcholine, and other neurotransmitters *(89)*.

EAAs

The high levels of extracellular EAAs normally seen following ischemia and TBI are associated with pathophysiologic widespread depolarization. EAA clearance from the synaptic cleft is by reuptake into the presynaptic bouton or into astrocytes, both of which are energy-dependent processes. Therefore, both the high levels of extracellular EAAs and the widespread depolarization seen following TBI or ischemia may be the result of failure of reuptake of EAAs *(90)*. In an animal model of global cerebral ischemia, Busto et al. *(56)* found that moderate hypothermia led to high interstitial concentrations of EAAs. Mitani et al. *(91)* found that brain temperature reductions of 2°C resulted in half the level of extracellular glutamate seen in normothermic controls. In human studies, patients with severe TBI had increasing CSF levels of glutamate for up to 96 h following initial injury *(46,92)*. In the study by Marion et al. *(22)*, patients with a GCS admission score of 5–7 demonstrated a significant reduction in CSF glutamate concentrations following treatment with moderate hypothermia ($p = 0.001$).

Posttraumatic Inflammatory Process

Cytokines, specifically interleukin-1β (IL-1β), have been found in elevated concentrations in ventricular CSF following TBI *(93,94)*. IL-1β is found primarily in macrophages in the peripheral blood, in activated astrocytes, and in microglia in the brain. It is thought to play an integral role in microvascular injury *(95,96)*. Vasodilatation, increased endothelial permeability, and initiation leukostasis and neutrophil activation are all consequences of pathologic release of cytokines such as IL-1β *(95–99)*. In a randomized clinical trial of hypothermia used for 24 h early after injury, a significant reduction of the CSF levels of IL-1β was found in the hypothermia group as compared to the normothermia group, both during the cooling phase and after the hypothermia patients were rewarmed ($p = 0.03$ for subgroup GCS 5–7) (**Table 3**) *(22)*. Recently, Kimura et al. *(100)* studied the effects of cooling on the white blood cell release of cytokines. In this in vitro study, cooling of stimulated peripheral mononuclear cells delayed the release of IL-1β, IL-6, and tumor necrosis factor (TNF) compared with cells kept normothermic after stimulation.

Extravasation of polymorphonuclear leukocytes (PMNs) in the area of injury occurs very early after injury in several different models of experimental TBI, and has been shown to correlate with the development of cerebral edema *(101,102)*. Early canine studies conducted by Rosomoff *(16,57)* demonstrated that treatment with hypothermia decreased the posttraumatic cellular inflammatory response incited by experimental head injury compared to normothermic controls. This effect of hypothermia is likely mediated by several mechanisms including preservation of the BBB, thereby limiting extravasation of inflammatory cells and mediators into the area of injury *(103)*, suppressing release of cytokines *(22)*, and reducing CBF.

BBB Permeability

Increased BBB permeability following ischemic injury may contribute to secondary brain injury by allowing the passage of ions, EAAs, neurotransmitters, and water. Several investigators have demonstrated that BBB permeability, following traumatic or ischemic injury, may be modulated by temperature (**Table 5**) *(104,105)*. Hypothermia has been shown to reduce the concentration of radiolabeled tracers across the BBB when compared to normothermic controls *(106)*. In addition, edema formation following controlled bilateral carotid artery occlusion in gerbils was significantly reduced in the animals treated with moderate hypothermia of 30–31°C *(59)*. Other investigators have shown that following global ischemia elevations in brain temperature to 39°C augment BBB permeability to tracer proteins *(107)*.

Intracellular Energy Stores

In ischemia models, hypothermia (32.5°C) was found to delay the depletion of ATP within the hippocampus. It is important to note that depletion of ATP stores was only retarded, but not prevented *(33)*. Other investigators found reductions in ATP loss when animals were cooled *(46,106)*. Delays in ATP depletion may provide early cerebral protection during brief ischemic insults or during the initial onset of brain injury.

COMPLICATIONS RESULTING FROM MODERATE HYPOTHERMIA

In the early clinical hypothermia studies, cooling was implicated as a cause for cardiac arrhythmias, coagulation disorders, blood sludging, and other medical problems primarily observed in patients cooled below 27°C. Hypothermia has also been shown to increase the risk of infections, most commonly pulmonary *(108,109)*. As demonstrated by Marion et al. *(22)*, patients with severe TBI managed with moderate hypothermia (32–33°C) for 24 h did not have more significant medical complications than normothermic controls. Although none of the recent clinical trials found an increased incidence of cardiac arrhythmias *(17,20–22)*, one study did detect a significant increase in the incidence of sepsis *(17)*. Furthermore, several Japanese studies have identified a significant risk of infections if patients are cooled for longer periods of time *(110,111)*.

Hypothermia has been shown to cause coagulopathies *(106)*. This hypothermic complication, however, is seen primarily when patients are cooled to temperatures less than 30°C *(106)*. In a phase II clinical study, Clifton et al. *(17)* showed an increase in the PT ($p < 0.001$) and partial thromboplastin time (PTT) ($p < 0.001$). Interestingly, prolonged coagulation parameters were not appreciated until hypothermia patients were in their rewarming or normothermic phases of treatment. During the cooling period, no significant differences were found in the PT or PTT between the hypothermia treated patients and those who were not cooled *(17)*. Oung et al. *(112)* utilized comparisons of template bleeding times in hypothermic and normothermic swine to investigate the effect of therapeutic moderate hypothermia on blood coagulation. They found a significant prolongation of the template bleeding time in pigs cooled to 30°C as compared with animals tested at 37°C.

Hypothermia-induced coagulopathy in patients with severe TBI has important clinical implications. In addition to the intracranial hemorrhages caused by their primary traumatic injury, these patients have a 20–30% incidence of delayed posttraumatic intracranial hemorrhage. However, at least one report found that treatment with moderate hypothermia did not result in increased rates of secondary delayed intracranial hemorrhages as compared to normothermic controls *(19)*.

SUMMARY

A large number of both clinical and experimental studies suggest that therapeutic moderate hypothermia (32–33°C) is an effective means of improving patient outcome following severe TBI. Hypothermia appears to mitigate several pathophysiologic mechanisms of secondary brain injury such as ischemia *(47)*, metabolic alterations, widespread depolarizations *(50)*, amino acid excitotoxicity, and vascular injury with disruption of the BBB *(54)*. Unchecked, these mechanisms of injury may lead to brain swelling, worsening ischemia, increased neuronal damage, and cell death.

As demonstrated by recent clinical trials, moderate hypothermia is a safe and effective method of reducing secondary brain injury *(28,63)*. Several studies suggest that mild to moderate hypothermia does not cause a significant increase in complications such as cardiac arrhythmias, coagulation disorders, blood sludging, or systemic infections. In the largest single-center study, a significant improvement in clinical outcome was demonstrated at 3, 6, and 12 mo after injury for those patients with an initial GCS of 5–7. Results from a multicenter trial of therapeutic moderate hypothermia for 48 h showed no benefit of hypothermia on neurologic outcome at 6 mo overall, but may have improved outcome in patients ≤ 45 yr old treated with hypothermia. The data suggest that hypothermia may be ineffective in patients who were normothermic on admission (>35°C). Hypothermia was beneficial in 30% of patients who were hypothermic on admission, but detrimental to patients older than 45 yr of age *(25)*. It should be noted that all groups demonstrated a reduction in ICP following treatment with hypothermia. Despite the disappointing results of this large clinical trial for TBI, two large prospective clinical trials of therapeutic moderate hypothermia for cardiac arrest have shown benefit with this therapy *(113,114)*.

Future multicenter clinical studies examining certain subgroups of patients may aid clinicians in selecting brain-injured patients that will benefit from therapeutic moderate hypothermia.

ACKNOWLEDGMENTS

This work was supported by a grant from the United States Public Health Service, National Institute of Neurological Disorders and Stroke—NS 30318.

REFERENCES

1. Fay T. (1943) Observations on generalized refrigeration in cases of severe cerebral trauma. *Assoc. Res. Nerv. Ment. Dis. Proc.* **24,** 611–619.
2. Hendrick E. B. (1959) The use of hypothermia in severe head injuries in childhood. *Ann. Surg.* **79,** 362–364.
3. Lazorthes G. and Campan L. (1958) Hypothermia in the treatment of craniocerebral traumatism. *J. Neurosurg.* **15,** 162–167.
4. Sedzimir C. B. (1959) Therapeutic hypothermia in cases of head injury. *J. Neurosurg.* **16,** 407–414.
5. Woringer E., Schneider J., Baumgartener J., and Thomalske G. (1954) Essai critique sur l'effet de l'hibernation artificielle sur 19 cas de souffrance du tronc cerebral apres traumatisme selectionnes pour leur gravite parmi 270 comas postcommotionels. *Anesth. Analg. (Paris)* **11,** 34–45.
6. Drake C. G. and Jory T. A. (1962) Hypothermia in the treatment of critical head injury. *Can. Med. Assoc. J.* **87,** 887–891.
7. Shapiro H. M., Wyte S. R., and Loeser J. (1974) Barbiturate-augmented hypothermia for reduction of persistent intracranial hypertension. *J. Neurosurg.* **40,** 90–100.
8. Mouritzen C. V. and Andersen M. N. (1966) Mechanisms of ventricular fibrillation during hypothermia: relative changes in myocardial refractory period and conduction velocity. *J. Thorac. Cardiovasc. Surg.* **51,** 585–589.
9. Rohrer M. J. and Natale A. M. (1992) Effect of hypothermia on the coagulation cascade. *Crit. Care Med.* **20,** 1402–1405.
10. Bailey C. P., Cookson B. A., Downing D. F., and Neptune W. B. (1954) Cardiac surgery under hypothermia. *J. Thorac. Surg.* **27,** 73–95.
11. Mohri H. and Merendino K. A. (1969) Hypothermia with or without a pump oxygenator. In *Surgery of the Chest* (Gibbon J. H., ed.), W. B. Saunders, Philadelphia, pp. 643–673.

12. Dietrich W. D., Alonso O., Busto R., Globus M. Y., and Ginsberg M. D. (1994) Posttraumatic brain hypothermia reduces histopathological damage following concussive brain injury in the rat. *Acta Neuropathol.* **87,** 250–258.

13. Sano T., Drummond J. C., Patel P. M., Grafe M. R., Watson J. C., and Cole D. J. (1992) A comparison of the cerebral protective effects of isoflurane and mild hypothermia in a model of incomplete forebrain ischemia in the rat. *Anesthesiology* **76,** 221–228.

14. Moyer D. J., Welsh F. A., and Zager E. L. (1992) Spontaneous cerebral hypothermia diminishes focal infarction in rat brain. *Stroke* **23,** 1812–1816.

15. Leonov Y., Sterz F., Safar P., et al. (1990) Mild cerebral hypothermia during and after cardiac arrest improves neurologic outcome in dogs. *J. Cereb. Blood Flow Metab.* **10,** 57–70.

16. Rosomoff H. L. (1966) Relationship of metabolism to hypothermia. *Res. Publ. Assoc.* **41,** 116–126.

17. Clifton G. L., Allen S., Barrodale P., et al. (1993) A phase II study of moderate hypothermia in severe brain injury. *J. Neurotrauma* **10,** 263–271; discussion 273.

18. Marion D. W., Obrist W. D., Carlier P. M., Penrod L. E., and Darby J. M. (1993) The use of moderate therapeutic hypothermia for patients with severe head injuries: a preliminary report. *J. Neurosurg.* **79,** 354–362.

19. Resnick D. K., Marion D. W., and Darby J. M. (1994) The effect of hypothermia on the incidence of delayed traumatic intracerebral hemorrhage. *Neurosurgery* **34,** 252–255; discussion 255–256.

20. Shiozaki T., Sugimoto H., Taneda M., et al. (1993) Effect of mild hypothermia on uncontrollable intracranial hypertension after severe head injury. *J. Neurosurg.* **79,** 363–368.

21. Metz C., Holzschuh M., Bein T., et al. (1996) Moderate hypothermia in patients with severe head injury: cerebral and extracerebral effects. *J. Neurosurg.* **85,** 533–541.

22. Marion D. W., Penrod L. E., Kelsey S. F., et al. (1997) Treatment of traumatic brain injury with moderate hypothermia. *N. Engl. J. Med.* **336,** 540–546.

23. Jiang J., Yu M., and Zhu C. (2000) Effect of long-term mild hypothermia therapy in patients with severe traumatic brain injury: 1-year follow-up review of 87 cases. *J. Neurosurg.* **93,** 546–549.

24. Marion D. W. (1997) Therapeutic moderate hypothermia for severe traumatic brain injury. *J. Intens. Care Med.* **12,** 239–248.

25. Clifton G. L., Miller E. R., Choi S. C., et al. (2001) Lack of effect of induction of hypothermia after acute brain injury. *N. Engl. J. Med.* **344,** 556–563.

26. Cairns C. J. and Andrews P. J. (2002) Management of hyperthermia in traumatic brain injury. *Curr. Opin. Crit. Care* **8,** 106–110.

27. Natale J. E., Joseph J. G., Helfaer M. A., and Shaffner D. H. (2000) Early hyperthermia after traumatic brain injury in children: risk factors, influence on length of stay, and effect on short-term neurologic status. *Crit. Care Med.* **28,** 2608–2615.

28. Marion D. W. (2001) Therapeutic moderate hypothermia and fever. *Curr. Pharm. Des.* **7,** 1533–1536.

29. Chatzipanteli K., Alonso O. F., Kraydieh S., and Dietrich W. D. (2000) Importance of posttraumatic hypothermia and hyperthermia on the inflammatory response after fluid percussion brain injury: biochemical and immunocytochemical studies. *J. Cereb. Blood Flow Metab.* **20,** 531–542.

30. Rossi S., Zanier E. R., Mauri I., Columbo A., and Stocchetti N. (2001) Brain temperature, body core temperature, and intracranial pressure in acute cerebral damage. *J. Neurol. Neurosurg. Psychiatry* **71,** 448–454.

31. Jiang J. Y., Gao G. Y., Li W. P., Yu M. K., and Zhu C. (2002) Early indicators of prognosis in 846 cases of severe traumatic brain injury. *J. Neurotrauma* **19,** 869–874.

32. Buchan A. and Pulsinelli W. A. (1990) Hypothermia but not the *N*-methyl-D-aspartate antagonist, MK-801, attenuates neuronal damage in gerbils subjected to transient global ischemia. *J. Neurosci.* **10,** 311–316.

33. Welsh F. A., Sims R. E., and Harris V. A. (1990) Mild hypothermia prevents ischemic injury in gerbil hippocampus. *J. Cereb. Blood Flow Metab.* **10,** 557–563.

34. Minamisawa H., Smith M. L., and Siesjo B. K. (1990) The effect of mild hyperthermia and hypothermia on brain damage following 5, 10, and 15 minutes of forebrain ischemia. *Ann. Neurol.* **28,** 26–33.

35. Clifton G. L., Jiang J. Y., Lyeth B. G., Jenkins L. W., Hamm R. J., and Hayes R. L. (1991) Marked protection by moderate hypothermia after experimental traumatic brain injury. *J. Cereb. Blood Flow Metab.* **11,** 114–121.

36. Busto R., Dietrich W. D., Globus M. Y., Valdes I., Scheinberg P., and Ginsberg M. D. (1987) Small differences in intraischemic brain temperature critically determine the extent of ischemic neuronal injury. *J. Cereb. Blood Flow Metab.* **7,** 729–738.

37. Busto R., Dietrich W. D., Globus M. Y., and Ginsberg M. D. (1989) Postischemic moderate hypothermia inhibits CA1 hippocampal ischemic neuronal injury. *Neurosci. Lett.* **101,** 299–304.

38. Clifton G. L., Taft W. C., Blair R. E., Choi S. C., and DeLorenzo R. J. (1989) Conditions for pharmacologic evaluation in the gerbil model of forebrain ischemia. *Stroke* **20,** 1545–1552.

39. Busto R., Dietrich W. D., Globus M. Y., and Ginsberg M. D. (1989) The importance of brain temperature in cerebral ischemic injury. *Stroke* **20,** 1113–1114.

40. Pomeranz S., Safar P., Radovsky A., Tisherman S. A., Alexander H., and Stezoski W. (1993) The effect of resuscitative moderate hypothermia following epidural brain compression on cerebral damage in a canine outcome model. *J. Neurosurg.* **79,** 241–251.

41. Marion D. W. and White M. J. (1996) Treatment of experimental brain injury with moderate hypothermia and 21- aminosteroids. *J. Neurotrauma* **13,** 139–147.

42. Lyeth B. G., Jiang J. Y., and Liu S. (1993) Behavioral protection by moderate hypothermia initiated after experimental traumatic brain injury. *J. Neurotrauma* **10,** 57–64.

43. Gordon C. J. (2001) The therapeutic potential of regulated hypothermia. *Emerg. Med. J.* **18,** 81–89.

44. Blumbergs P. C., Jones N. R., and North J. B. (1989) Diffuse axonal injury in head trauma. *J. Neurol. Neurosurg. Psychiatry* **52,** 838–841.

45. Erb D. E. and Povlishock J. T. (1988) Axonal damage in severe traumatic brain injury: an experimental study in cat. *Acta Neuropathol.* **76,** 347–358.

46. Baker A. J., Moulton R. J., MacMillan V. H., and Shedden P. M. (1993) Excitatory amino acids in cerebrospinal fluid following traumatic brain injury in humans. *J. Neurosurg.* **79,** 369–372.

47. Jennett W. B. (1970) Secondary ischaemic brain damage after head injury. *J. Clin. Pathol. Suppl.* **4,** 172–175.

48. Michenfelder J. D. and Theye R. A. (1970) The effects of anesthesia and hypothermia on canine cerebral ATP and lactate during anoxia produced by decapitation. *Anesthesiology* **33,** 430–439.

49. Michenfelder J. D. (1988) The hypothermic brain. In *Anesthesia and the Brain: Clinical, Functional, Metabolic and Vascular Correlates* (Michenfelder J. D., ed.), Churchill Livingstone, New York.

50. Hayes R. L., Stonnington H. H., Lyeth B. G., Dixon C. E., and Yamamoto T. (1986) Metabolic and neurophysiologic sequelae of brain injury: a cholinergic hypothesis. *Cent. Nerv. Syst. Trauma* **3,** 163–173.

51. Benveniste H. (1991) The excitotoxin hypothesis in relation to cerebral ischemia. *Cerebrovasc. Brain Metab. Rev.* **3,** 213–245.

52. Choi D. W. and Rothman S. M. (1990) The role of glutamate neurotoxicity in hypoxic–ischemic neuronal death. *Annu. Rev. Neurosci.* **13,** 171–182.

53. Faden A. I., Demediuk P., Panter S. S., and Vink R. (1989) The role of excitatory amino acids and NMDA receptors in traumatic brain injury. *Science* **244,** 798–800.

54. Povlishock J. T. and Lyeth B. G. (1989) Traumatically induced blood–brain barrier disruption: a conduit for the passage of circulating excitatory neurotransmitters. *Soc. Neurosci. Abstr.* **15,** 1113 (Abstr).

55. Wei E. P., Kontos H. A., Dietrich W. D., Povlishock J. T., and Ellis E. F. (1981) Inhibition by free radical scavengers and by cyclooxygenase inhibitors of pial arteriolar abnormalities from concussive brain injury in cats. *Circ. Res.* **48,** 95–103.

56. Busto R., Globus M. Y., Dietrich W. D., Martinez E., Valdes I., and Ginsberg M. D. (1989) Effect of mild hypothermia on ischemia-induced release of neurotransmitters and free fatty acids in rat brain. *Stroke* **20,** 904–910.

57. Rosomoff H. L. (1959) Experimental brain injury during hypothermia. *J. Neurosurg.* **16,** 177–187.

58. Rosomoff H. L., Shulman K., and Raynor R. (1960) Experimental brain injury and delayed hypothermia. *Surg. Gynecol. Obstet.* **110,** 27–32.

59. Dempsey R. J., Combs D. J., Maley M. E., Cowen D. E., Roy M. W., and Donaldson D. L. (1987) Moderate hypothermia reduces postischemic edema development and leukotriene production. *Neurosurgery* **21,** 177–181.

60. Lei B., Tan X., Cai H., Xu Q., and Guo Q. (1994) Effect of moderate hypothermia on lipid peroxidation in canine brain tissue after cardiac arrest and resuscitation. *Stroke* **25,** 147–152.

61. Lyeth B. G., Jiang J. Y., Robinson S. E., Guo H., and Jenkins L. W. (1993) Hypothermia blunts acetylcholine increase in CSF of traumatically brain injured rats. *Mol. Chem. Neuropathol.* **18,** 247–256.

62. Taft W. C., Yang K., Dixon C. E., Clifton G. L., and Hayes R. L. (1993) Hypothermia attenuates the loss of hippocampal microtubule-associated protein 2 (MAP2) following traumatic brain injury. *J. Cereb. Blood Flow Metab.* **13,** 796–802.

63. Bayir H., Clark R. S., and Kochanek P. M. (2003) Promising strategies to minimize secondary brain injury after head trauma. *Crit. Care Med.* **31,** S112–117.

64. Meyer J. S., Kondo A., Nomura F., Sakamoto K., and Teraura T. (1970) Cerebral hemodynamics and metabolism following experimental head injury. *J. Neurosurg.* **32,** 304–319.

65. Sood S. C., Gulati S. C., Kumar M., and Kak V. K. (1980) Cerebral metabolism following brain injury. II. Lactic acid changes. *Acta Neurochir.* **53,** 47–51.

66. Bouma G. J., Muizelaar J. P., Choi S. C., Newlon P. G., and Young H. F. (1991) Cerebral circulation and metabolism after severe traumatic brain injury: the elusive role of ischemia. *J. Neurosurg.* **75,** 685–693.

67. Bouma G. J., Muizelaar J. P., Stringer W. A., Choi S. C., Fatouros P., and Young H. F. (1992) Ultra-early evaluation of regional cerebral blood flow in severely head-injured patients using xenon-enhanced computerized tomography. *J. Neurosurg.* **77,** 360–368.

68. Marion D. W., Darby J., and Yonas H. (1991) Acute regional cerebral blood flow changes caused by severe head injuries. *J. Neurosurg.* **74,** 407–414.

69. Bullock R., Inglis F. M., Kuroda Y., Butcher S., McCulloch J., and Maxwell W. (1991) Transient hippocampal hypermetabolism associated with glutamate release after acute subdural haematoma in the rat: a potentially neurotoxic mechanism? *J. Cereb. Blood Flow Metab.* **11,** S109 (Abstr).

70. Kuroda Y., Inglis F. M., Miller J. D., McCulloch J., Graham D. I., and Bullock R. (1992) Transient glucose hypermetabolism after acute subdural hematoma in the rat. *J. Neurosurg.* **76,** 471–477.

71. Miller J. D., Bullock R., Graham D. I., Chen M. H., and Teasdale G. M. (1990) Ischemic brain damage in a model of acute subdural hematoma. *Neurosurgery* **27,** 433–439.

72. Stone H. H., Donnelly C., and Frobese A. S. (1956) The effect of lowered body temperature on the cerebral hemodynamics and metabolism of man. *Surg. Gynecol. Obstet.* **103,** 313–322.

73. Bering E. A. (1961) Effect of body temperature change on cerebral oxygen consumption of the intact monkey. *Am. J. Physiol.* **200,** 417–419.

74. Bigelow W. G., Lindsay W. K., and Greenwood W. F. (1950) Hypothermia. Its possible role in cardiac surgery: an investigation of factors governing survival in dogs at low body temperatures. *Ann. Surg.* **132,** 849–866.

75. McCulloch J., Savaki H. E., Jehle J., and Sokoloff L. (1982) Local cerebral glucose utilization in hypothermic and hyperthermic rats. *J. Neurochem.* **39,** 255–258.

76. Yoshino A., Hovda D. A., Kawamata T., Katayama Y., and Becker D. P. (1991) Dynamic changes in local cerebral glucose utilization following cerebral conclusion in rats: evidence of a hyper- and subsequent hypometabolic state. *Brain Res.* **561,** 106–119.

77. Kawamata T., Katayama Y., Hovda D. A., Yoshino A., and Becker D. P. (1992) Administration of excitatory amino acid antagonists via microdialysis attenuates the increase in glucose utilization seen following concussive brain injury. *J. Cereb. Blood Flow Metab.* **12,** 12–24.

78. Hagerdal M., Harp J., Nilsson L., and Siesjo B. K. (1975) The effect of induced hypothermia upon oxygen consumption in the rat brain. *J. Neurochem.* **24,** 311–316.

79. Rosomoff H. L. and Holaday D. A. (1954) Cerebral blood flow and cerebral oxygen consumption during hypothermia. *Am. J. Physiol.* **179,** 85–88.

80. Kuluz J. W., Prado R., Chang J., Ginsberg M. D., Schleien C. L., and Busto R. (1993) Selective brain cooling increases cortical cerebral blood flow in rats. *Am. J. Physiol.* **265,** H824–827.

81. Warner D. S., Deshpande J. K., and Wieloch T. (1986) The effect of isoflurane on neuronal necrosis following near-complete forebrain ischemia in the rat. *Anesthesiology* **64,** 19–23.

82. Gelb A. W., Boisvert D. P., Tang C., et al. (1989) Primate brain tolerance to temporary focal cerebral ischemia during isoflurane- or sodium nitroprusside-induced hypotension. *Anesthesiology* **70,** 678–683.

83. Michenfelder J. D. (1988) *Anesthesia and the Brain: Clinical, Functional, Metabolic and Vascular Correlates.* Churchill Livingstone, New York.

84. Kahveci F. S., Kahveci N., Alkan T., Goren B., Korfali E., and Ozluk K. (2001) Propofol versus isoflurane anesthesia under hypothermic conditions: effects on intracranial pressure and local cerebral blood flow after diffuse traumatic brain injury in the rat. *Surg. Neurol.* **56,** 206–214.

85. Siesjo B. K. (1992) Pathophysiology and treatment of focal cerebral ischemia. Part II: Mechanisms of damage and treatment. *J. Neurosurg.* **77,** 337–354.

86. Siesjo B. K. (1992) Pathophysiology and treatment of focal cerebral ischemia. Part I: Pathophysiology. *J. Neurosurg.* **77,** 169–184.

87. Siesjo B. K. (1981) Cell damage in the brain: a speculative synthesis. *J. Cereb. Blood Flow Metab.* **1,** 155–185.

88. Mitani A., Kadoya F., and Kataoka K. (1991) Temperature dependence of hypoxia-induced calcium accumulation in gerbil hippocampal slices. *Brain Res.* **562,** 159–163.

89. Katayama Y., Becker D. P., Tamura T., and Hovda D. A. (1990) Massive increases in extracellular potassium and the indiscriminate release of glutamate following concussive brain injury. *J. Neurosurg.* **73,** 889–900.

90. Swanson R. A., Chen J., and Graham S. H. (1994) Glucose can fuel glutamate uptake in ischemic brain. *J. Cereb. Blood Flow Metab.* **14,** 1–6.

91. Mitani A. and Kataoka K. (1991) Critical levels of extracellular glutamate mediating gerbil hippocampal delayed neuronal death during hypothermia: brain microdialysis study. *Neuroscience* **42,** 661–670.

92. Palmer A. M., Marion D. W., Botscheller M. L., Bowen D. M., and DeKosky S. T. (1994) Increased transmitter amino acid concentration in human ventricular CSF after brain trauma. *NeuroReport* **6,** 153–156.

93. McClain C. J., Cohen D., Ott L., Dinarello C. A., and Young B. (1987) Ventricular fluid interleukin-1 activity in patients with head injury. *J. Lab. Clin. Med.* **110,** 48–54.

94. Young A. B., Ott L. G., Beard D., Dempsey R. J., Tibbs P. A., and McClain C. J. (1988) The acute-phase response of the brain-injured patient. *J. Neurosurg.* **69,** 375–380.

95. Benveniste E. N. (1994) Cytokine circuits in brain. Implications for AIDS dementia complex. *Res. Publ. Assoc. Res. Nerv. Ment. Dis.* **72,** 71–88.

96. Giulian D., Baker T. J., Shih L. C., and Lachman L. B. (1986) Interleukin 1 of the central nervous system is produced by ameboid microglia. *J. Exp. Med.* **164,** 594–604.

97. Bevilacqua M. P., Pober J. S., Wheeler M. E., Cotran R. S., and Gimbrone M. A., Jr. (1985) Interleukin 1 acts on cultured human vascular endothelium to increase the adhesion of polymorphonuclear leukocytes, monocytes, and related leukocyte cell lines. *J. Clin. Invest.* **76,** 2003–2011.

98. Pober J. S., Gimbrone M. A., Jr., Lapierre L. A., et al. (1986) Overlapping patterns of activation of human endothelial cells by interleukin 1, tumor necrosis factor, and immune interferon. *J. Immunol.* **137,** 1893–1896.

99. Mantovani A. and Dejana E. (1987) Modulation of endothelial function by interleukin-1. A novel target for pharmacological intervention? *Biochem. Pharmacol.* **36,** 301–305.

100. Kimura A., Sakurada S., Ohkuni H., Todome Y., and Kurata K. (2002) Moderate hypothermia delays proinflammatory cytokine production of human peripheral blood mononuclear cells. *Crit. Care Med.* **30,** 1499–1502.

101. Clark R. S., Schiding J. K., Kaczorowski S. L., Marion D. W., and Kochanek P. M. (1994) Neutrophil accumulation after traumatic brain injury in rats: comparison of weight drop and controlled cortical impact models. *J. Neurotrauma* **11,** 499–506.

102. Dietrich W. D., Alonso O., Halley M., and Busto R. (1996) Delayed posttraumatic brain hyperthermia worsens outcome after fluid percussion brain injury: a light and electron microscopic study in rats. *Neurosurgery* **38,** 533–541; discussion 541.

103. Smith S. L. and Hall E. D. (1996) Mild pre- and posttraumatic hypothermia attenuates blood–brain barrier damage following controlled cortical impact injury in the rat. *J. Neurotrauma* **13,** 1–9.

104. Jiang J. Y., Lyeth B. G., Kapasi M. Z., Jenkins L. W., and Povlishock J. T. (1992) Moderate hypothermia reduces blood–brain barrier disruption following traumatic brain injury in the rat. *Acta Neuropathol.* **84,** 495–500.

105. Jiang J. Y., Lyeth B. G., Clifton G. L., Jenkins L. W., Hamm R. J., and Hayes R. L. (1991) Relationship between body and brain temperature in traumatically brain-injured rodents. *J. Neurosurg.* **74,** 492–496.

106. Krantis A. (1983) Hypothermia-induced reduction in the permeation of radiolabelled tracer substances across the blood–brain barrier. *Acta Neuropathol.* **60,** 61–69.

107. Dietrich W. D., Busto R., Halley M., and Valdes I. (1990) The importance of brain temperature in alterations of the blood–brain barrier following cerebral ischemia. *J. Neuropathol. Exp. Neurol.* **49,** 486–497.

108. Dripps R. D. (1956) *The Physiology of Induced Hypothermia.* National Academy of Sciences, Washington, D.C.

109. Steen P. A., Milde J. H., and Michenfelder J. D. (1980) The detrimental effects of prolonged hypothermia and rewarming in the dog. *Anesthesiology* **52,** 224–230.

110. Ishikawa K., Tanaka H., Shiozaki T., et al. (2000) Characteristics of infection and leukocyte count in severely head-injured patients treated with mild hypothermia. *J. Trauma* **49,** 912–922.

111. Shiozaki T., Hayakata T., Taneda M., et al. (2001) A multicenter prospective randomized controlled trial of the efficacy of mild hypothermia for severely head injured patients with low intracranial pressure. Mild Hypothermia Study Group in Japan. *J. Neurosurg.* **94,** 50–54.

112. Oung C. M., Li M. S., Shum-Tim D., Chiu R. C., and Hinchey E. J. (1993) In vivo study of bleeding time and arterial hemorrhage in hypothermic versus normothermic animals. *J. Trauma* **35,** 251–254.

113. Bernard S. A., Gray T. W., Buist M. D., et al. (2002) Treatment of comatose survivors of out-of-hospital cardiac arrest with induced hypothermia. *N. Engl. J. Med.* **346,** 557–563.

114. No author names available. (2002) The hypothermia after cardiac arrest study group: mild therapeutic hypothermia to improve the neurologic outcome after cardiac arrest. *N. Engl. J. Med.* **346,** 549–556.

9

Hypothermia

Clinical Experience in Stroke Patients

Stefan Schwab, MD,
and Werner Hacke, MD

CLINICAL EVIDENCE FOR THE IMPORTANCE OF BODY TEMPERATURE IN STROKE

In the last few years it has become increasingly evident that moderate hyperthermia, when present after brain ischemia or trauma, exacerbates the degree of resulting neuronal injury. Several recent clinical studies emphasized the importance of body temperature for stroke prognosis and severity. Azzimondi et al. *(1)* showed that fever in the first 7 d after stroke was an independent predictor of poor outcome. Out of 183 patients with acute ischemic or hemorrhagic stroke, fever occurred in 43% during the first week in hospital. Higher fever was associated with a worse prognosis, and patients with high fever were more likely to die within the first 10 d after stroke than those with lower temperatures. Reith et al. *(2)* demonstrated lower mortality and better outcome in patients with mild hypothermia (<36.5°C) on admission. The Copenhagen group classified 390 patients who were admitted within the first 6 h after stroke onset in three admission-temperature groups: hypothermic (<36.5°C), normothermic (>36.5–37.5°C), and hyperthermic (>37.5°C). By multiple regression analysis they found body temperature on admission to be highly correlated with clinical outcome and infarct size. The relationship between body temperature and poor outcome was independent of stroke severity on admission. A recent study from Davalos et al. *(3)* emphasized those findings, while they showed that patients with increased body temperatures on admission more often had an early neurological deterioration that led to a significantly worse outcome. The same group showed that a possible

From: *Hypothermia and Cerebral Ischemia: Mechanisms and Clinical Applications*
Edited by: C. M. Maier and G. K. Steinberg © Humana Press Inc., Totowa, NJ

mechanism for these findings was increased levels of glutamate measured in those patients who were hyperthermic *(4)*.

Other groups have emphasized that previous infections are an independent risk factor for acute stroke. This phenomenon might be at least in part attributable to the activation of cytokines and adhesion molecules such as the vascular cell adhesion molecule (VCAM) and intercellular adhesion molecule (ICAM) *(5)*.

STUDIES ON BRAIN TEMPERATURE IN STROKE AND OTHER DISEASES

Measurement of Brain Temperature: Where and How?

Interest in brain temperature monitoring has increased further with the emerging therapeutic potential of hypothermia as a neuroprotective measure. Although monitoring global brain temperature would be ideal, brain temperature probes can measure only in small areas of the brain. Until now, there has been no substitute for intraparenchymatous temperature monitoring. Several studies used bladder, tympanic membrane, esophagus, and pulmonary artery temperature measures to correlate with brain temperature. However, all these measurement sites did not reflect brain temperature exactly *(6–9)*.

Most of the previous studies on brain temperature monitoring were performed in neurosurgical patients with head trauma, brain tumor, or large intracerebral hematoma. Busto *(10)* addressed the importance of brain temperature in experimental cerebral ischemic injury. He was able to show a reduction in ischemic injury depending on the level of intraischemic brain temperatures.

For clinical practice other measurement sites to estimate brain temperature were evaluated. Conflicting results exist regarding jugular vein temperature recordings *(7–9)*. Two studies concluded that jugular venous temperatures are not a substitute for brain temperature following head trauma or cerebral ischemia *(8,9)*. These studies suggest that only invasive monitoring of intraparenchymatous temperature is reliable, but even within the brain significant temperature gradients were described. Depending on the depth of insertion, brain temperature was shown to vary 1°C or more *(6)*.

Does Body Core Temperature Reflect Brain Temperature?

In a study on brain temperature in patients with severe middle cerebral artery (MCA) infarction a significant gradient between brain tem-

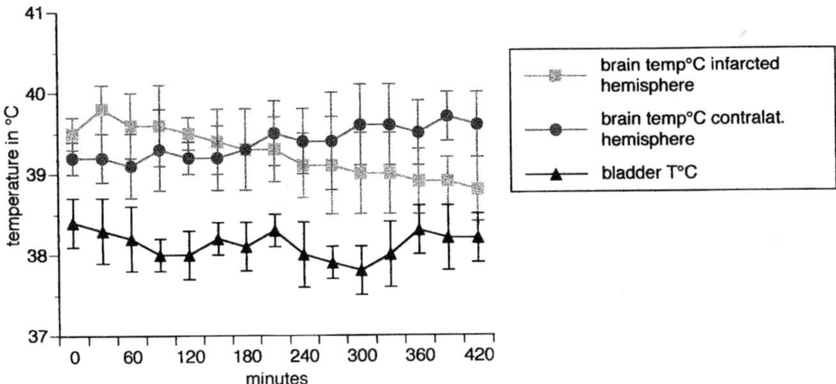

Fig. 1. Bilateral intraparenchymatous temperature monitoring with representative bladder temperatures in patients showing higher temperatures in the infarcted hemisphere within the first hours after stroke. Monitoring began within 6 h after onset of symptoms. Measurements were taken every 30 min.

perature and body core temperatures was observed. Not only was the disparity between body temperature and brain temperature established, but also a temperature gradient between infarcted and healthy hemispheres in the early phase of ischemia was demonstrated. Initially, temperatures in the infarcted hemisphere exceeded those of the healthy hemisphere by up to 0.8°C (**Fig. 1**) *(11)*.

These results confirm the findings of Mellergard and others, who showed a significant gradient between body core and brain temperatures in head trauma patients *(12,13)*. The explanation for this may be the high metabolic activity of cerebral tissue with a considerable production of heat *(14,15)*. Nurse and Corbett postulated an acute phase of locomotor hyperactivity to be the cause of a secondary temperature rise after experimental ischemia in a rat model *(14)*. A similar explanation is possible for the astonishing finding of initially increased temperatures in the infarcted hemisphere compared to the contralateral hemisphere in the first hours after ischemia. We can only speculate that this finding is the result of a release of excitatory neurotransmitters and increased energy (ATP) depletion and lactate accumulation during ischemia *(15–18)*. Another possibility is that in the early stages of infarct formation, a decrease in cerebral blood flow may result in a decreased capacity for the blood to carry off heat generated by local cerebral metabolism. In all recent clinical studies both in neurosurgical and in stroke patients, body temperature measurement did not adequately reflect brain temperature: with normothermic core temperatures, brain temperatures of 38°C and greater were measured. A better characterization of human brain temperature is necessary if hypothermia is to be implemented as a therapeutic tool *(19)*. However, brain temperature monitoring is safe and seems to bear no additional risk, compared to the intracranial pressure (ICP) devices routinely used in patients with intracranial hypertension.

METHODS TO CONTROL TEMPERATURE IN STROKE PATIENTS

Experimental data demonstrated that body temperature and brain temperature could differ significantly *(20)*. In accordance with these findings as described in the preceding, several authors reported a temperature gradient within the brain and between body core and brain in neurosurgical patients. For optimal use of hypothermia as a therapeutic tool for neuroprotection, methods for both continuous monitoring of brain temperature and for easy and readily available brain cooling are necessary. In animal models various measures of controlling brain temperature, including fanning, nasopharyngeal cooling, cardiopulmonary bypass, ice water immersion, or simply packing the head in ice have been employed *(19,21–25)*.

To date several methods have been used for induction and maintenance of clinical hypothermia. This includes body surface cooling with water blankets, cooled air fans, installation of cold gastric lavage, or transvascular cooling methods. A neurosurgical study used an extracorporal heat exchanger by which a cooling rate of 3.5°C per hour was achieved *(19)*. Within a mean of 1 h and 53 min brain temperature was decreased to 32°C. The advantages of this method are twofold. First, it allows a gradual and controlled rewarming, and second it is by far the most rapid cooling method used in all clinical studies. Metz and others achieved cooling head trauma patients to 33°C within 2.3–4.5 h *(26)*. Kurz reached body temperatures of 32°C within 3.6–4.8 h with cool air fanning *(27)*. The most important issue for the cooling velocity thereby was the incidence of thermoregulatory vasoconstriction. Until recently, the only rapidly available cooling method that was also easy to implement in stroke patients was external cooling. However, recent technological advances have led to the development of transvenous catheter devices that seem to safely achieve rapid cooling of patients *(28–31)*.

CLINICAL EXPERIENCE
WITH HYPOTHERMIA FOLLOWING STROKE

Definition of Hypothermia

Hypothermia has been used for thousands of years. The ancient Egyptians used hypothermia to treat fever. Hypothermic operations by physicians who were in Napoleon's army during the Prussian war in 1807 have been reported.

The normal body temperature is usually considered 37°C, even though there is a significant diurnal variation, up to 0.6°C. Body core temperature can be measured at varying sites. The shell temperatures are measured as sublingual, axillary, or as skin temperatures. Core temperatures reflect tympanic membrane, esophageal, rectal, bladder, and pulmonary artery measurements. Hypothermia was defined as mild (34°C), moderate (28°C), and deep (below 28°C) *(32)*. The methods to induce hypothermia varied from ice water immersion to application of ice packs, cooling helmets, and so forth. Systemic oxygen demand decreases with falling core temperatures. Corresponding to this, a drop in carbon dioxide production, plasma potassium, and carbohydrate metabolism is seen. Hypothermia reduces both the cerebral demand needed for neuronal activity and the energy requirements necessary for intrinsic cellular support and membrane homeostasis. Additional mechanisms of cerebral protection include decreased glutamate and dopamine release, lowering of ICP, and altered expression of genes involved in programmed cell death (apoptosis) *(18)*.

COURSE AND PROGNOSIS
OF MALIGNANT MCA INFARCTS

So called "malignant" MCA stroke presents clinically with a severe hemispheric stroke syndrome that includes hemiplegia, forced eye and head deviation, and progressive deterioration of consciousness within the first 2 d *(33)*. Thereafter, unilateral pupillary dilatation occurs within 2–4 d after onset of symptoms. ICP measurements frequently exceed 30 mmHg. Although unilateral pupillary dilatation may initially be reversible, it almost always indicates death due to herniation, despite maximum medical treatment of brain edema. When this clinical presentation is accompanied by early computed tomography (CT) signs of major infarct during the first 12 h after stroke and a distal intracerebral artery (ICA) or proximal MCA (+ACA) occlusion, massive hemispheric swelling occurs during the next 24–72 h. The prognosis is poor for complete MCA territory stroke and the mortality rate as high as 80%.

THERAPEUTIC OPTIONS IN MALIGNANT MCA INFARCTS

Conventional treatment of raised ICP in this condition consists of artificial ventilation, osmotherapy, and barbiturate administration. The value and duration of these measures has come under scrutiny. Prolonged hyperventilation has been discouraged, as the potential decrease in cerebral arterial blood flow resulting from additional hypocarbia might exacerbate tissue ischemia *(34)*. Early use of agents such as glycerol or mannitol, at least in theory, may actually hasten tissue shifts and therefore lead to an aggravation of brain edema *(35)*. Barbiturate therapy has to date failed to prove to be of therapeutic benefit in the treatment of postischemic brain edema *(36)*.

Decompressive surgery for control of otherwise intractable, elevated ICP was proposed for a variety of neurological disorders such as head trauma, space-occupying hemispheric infarction, or subdural hematoma. The surgical management of intracranial hypertension is directed at improving cerebral perfusion, and preventing ischemic damage and mechanical compression of the brain against various intracranial structures such as the falx, tentorium, or the sphenoid ridge. However, especially in patients with cerebrovascular accidents, there is still controversy as to when and how to implement this invasive therapeutical procedure *(37)*. Because of the potential adverse effects of "conventional medical therapy" and the disparity regarding when to initiate a neurosurgical intervention, new therapeutic concepts for the treatment of ischemic brain edema have been considered.

HYPOTHERMIA IN MALIGNANT MCA INFARCTS

It is known from animal models with global ischemia and traumatic brain injury that moderate hypothermia attenuates secondary brain damage by reducing cerebral ischemia and postischemic brain edema and preserving the blood–brain barrier. Even though hypothermia has potent cerebroprotective effects after experimental focal ischemia, clinical studies on hypothermic therapy after MCA infarction were not available until recently. We performed a pilot study investigating the efficacy, feasibility, and safety of induced moderate hypothermia in the therapy of patients with acute, severe MCA infarction and increased ICP.

Table 1
Protocol for Delivery of Mild Hypothermia in Stroke Patients

- All patients are ventilated and sedated (for sedation use fentanyl and propofol).
- Prior to initiation of hypothermia insert a Foley catheter for bladder temperature monitoring.
- All patients are subjected to ICP monitoring with a temperature-monitoring device.
- To prevent shivering use neuromuscular blockers via an infusion pump (Atracrium 200 mg in 50 mL).
- Induce hypothermia with cooling catheter.
- For initiation use also alcohol washing of the whole body.
- Aim for a temperature decline of 1.5°C/h.
- Hypothermia of 33°C is maintained for 48–72 h.
- Thereafter stop active cooling and begin slowly active rewarming (0.1°C/h).
- At 36°C stop neuromuscular blockers.

Temperature Protocol

Brain temperature was measured with the Spiegelberg intraparenchymatous ICP probe, which has a thermistor in its tip. The accuracy for the temperature measurements is <0.1°C. A Foley temperature catheter for bladder temperature reading with a temperature resolution of 0.1°C was used for monitoring of body core temperature (Mon-a-therm™, Mallinckrodt, St. Louis, MO, USA). All patients were sedated with fentanyl and propofol and received neuromuscular blockade with continuous infusion of atracurium (0.3–0.6 mg/kg i.v.). The room temperature in the intensive care unit was between 18°C and 20°C. In this study, cooling blankets (Polar Bair™, Augustine Medical, Eden Prairie, MN, USA) with cool ventilator air fanning the patients' body surfaces were used for external cooling. Acid–base management was guided by blood gas analysis not corrected for temperature to maintain autoregulation *(32)*. Once the body core temperature reached 33°C, it was kept between 33° and 34°C for 48–72 h. During the next 24 h the patient was passively rewarmed to a normal temperature (**Table 1**).

Results for Hypothermic Therapy

We studied 30 patients with malignant MCA infarction, who were treated with moderate hypothermia of 33°C with a mean delay of 14 h after onset of symptoms. The time required for cooling to 33°C bladder

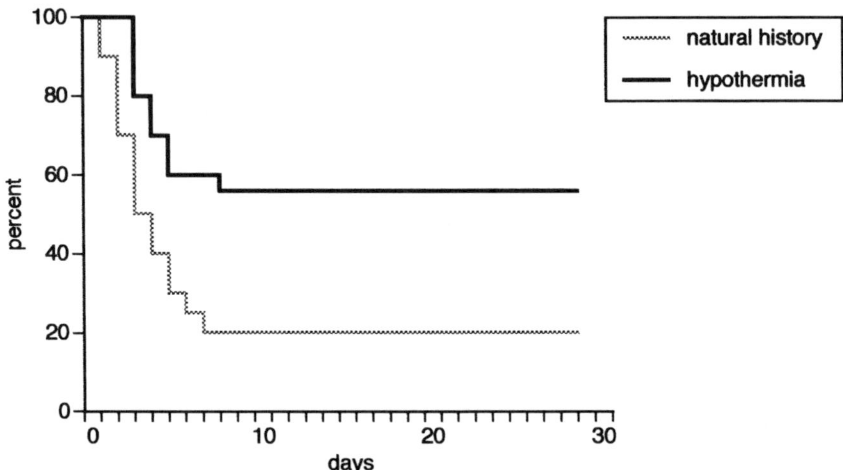

Fig. 2. Survival curve of all patients treated with moderate hypothermia vs patients treated with conventional therapy 33.

temperature lasted from 3.5 to 6.2 h. Moderate hypothermia was sustained for 48–72 h (median 65 h). Passive rewarming took between 17 and 24 h (median 18 h). All patients in this study fulfilled the criteria for diagnosis of a "malignant" MCA infarction *(33)*. However, the mortality was only 43% (13/30) and the survivors reached a favorable outcome with a mean Barthel index of 70 (**Fig. 2**).

A significant reduction of the ICP was seen, which was similar to the results of Marion and Shiozaki, who used hypothermic therapy in traumatic brain injuries *(37,38)*. With an unaffected mean arterial blood pressure (MABP) and increased cerebral perfusion pressure (CPP), hypothermic therapy appeared to benefit stroke patients, as uncontrolled intracranial hypertension is the main cause of death in the first week after stroke. However, rewarming the patients consistently led to a secondary rise of ICP, which required additional ICP therapy with mannitol. In some cases it even exaggerated the initial ICP levels (**Fig. 3**).

It is known that the rewarming period is a high-risk time for brain injury because metabolic needs may outstrip oxygen delivery at various temperatures *(39)*. In the 13 patients who died, nine had untreatable elevation of ICP during rewarming, while in six patients, signs of transtentorial herniation occurred with a body temperature of 33°C. The rebound increase in ICP after rewarming might suggest that hypothermia only delays the deleterious effects caused by ischemic injury, therefore not resulting in any substantial improvement. The fact that the

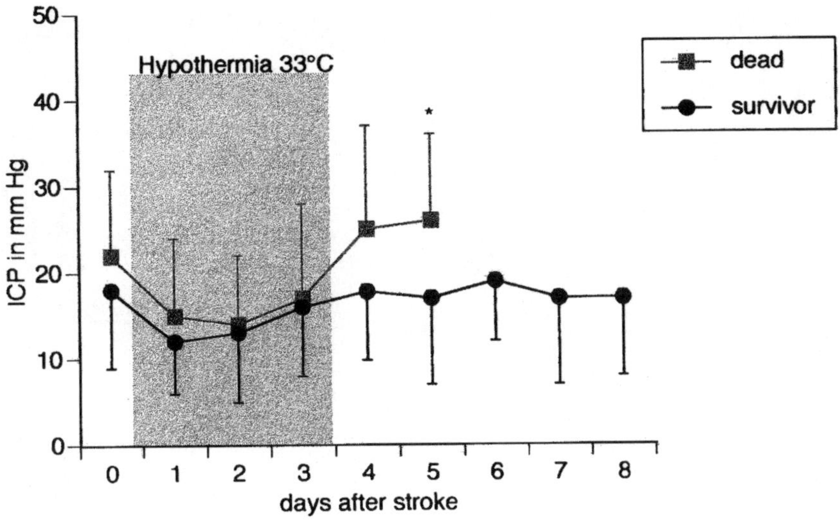

Fig. 3. Time course of daily maximum ICP values in those patients who survived and those who subsequently died treated with hypothermia (*$p < 0.05$).

Table 2
**Effects of Moderate Hypothermia
on Intracranial and on Systemic Physiologic Characteristics**

Variable	Normothermia	Hypothermia	After rewarming
ICP (mmHg)	20.9 ± 12.4	13.4 ± 8.3^a	19.4 ± 8.7
CPP (mmHg)	68 ± 14	78 ± 21^a	70 ± 21
Brain temperature (°C)	38.4 ± 1.3	33.3 ± 0.7	37.4 ± 0.9
Body temperature (°C)	37.5 ± 0.9	33.0 ± 0.2	36.8 ± 0.9
Heart rate (bpm)	84 ± 6	62 ± 10^a	80 ± 12

ICP, Intracranial pressure; CPP, cerebral perfusion pressure.
[a]$p < 0.05$ compared to baseline value.

majority of patients had lower ICP levels than before induction of hypothermia argues clearly against this hypothesis (**Table 2** and **Fig. 4**).

However, rewarming has to be considered as the "critical phase" of hypothermic therapy. This rebound intracranial hypertension after rewarming might be due to a proposed hypermetabolic response after induced hypothermia, as it was described after cardiopulmonary bypass surgery *(40)*.

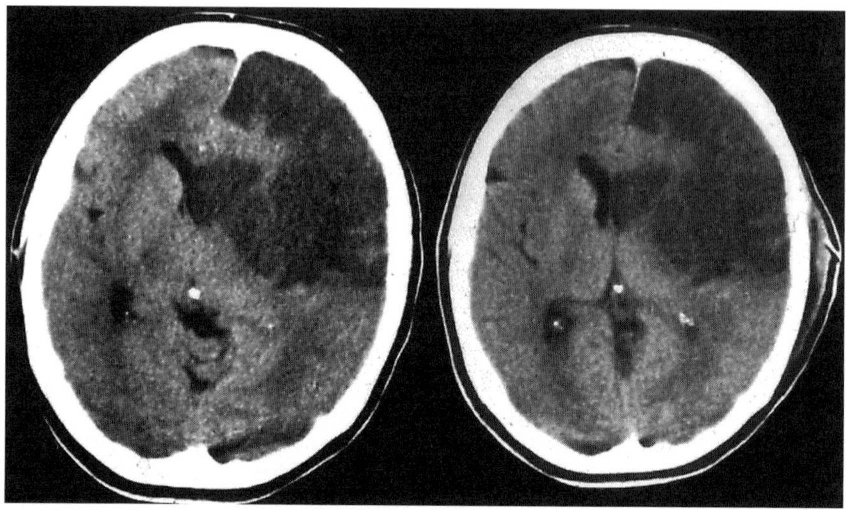

Fig. 4. (a) CT scan at the septum pellucidum level in a 35-yr-old woman with left hemispheric MCA infarction. Note compression of the lateral ventricle and severe midline shift (5 mm). (b) After 12 h of hypothermic therapy reduction of mass effect and only slight midline shift (2 mm).

RISKS OF HYPOTHERMIA

Complications of hypothermia are numerous and can be life threatening. The extent of hypothermia is limited by ventricular ectopy and fibrillation. Below 32°C prolongation of the P–R interval and QRS complex will occur. It is followed by an increased Q–T interval, and finally below 27°C ventricular fibrillation may occur. Electrolyte disorders may be one of the mechanisms through which hypothermia can cause arrhythmias. Abiki et al. *(41)* reported the occurrence of hypophosphatemia in 15 patients with brain injury who were treated with hypothermia (32–33°C, 3- to 4-d duration). Besides these cardiac side effects, hematologic perturbations are often seen, primarily thrombocytopenia and clotting disturbances. Abnormalities in clotting mechanisms occur by slowing the enzyme-mediated cascade and by promoting fibrinolysis (**Table 3**).

In several animal studies severe adverse effects of hypothermia were clotting abnormalities and coagulopathy *(22,42)*. In baboons, systemic hypothermia led to increased bleeding times *(43)*. In men the enzymatic reactions of the coagulation cascade were shown to be strongly inhibited by hypothermia *(44,45)*. However, severe clotting abnormalities have

Table 3
Side Effects of Moderate Hypothermia on Various Organ Systems

Variable	Normothermia	Hypothermia	After rewarming
Platelet count (cts/nL)	183 (145–310)	110 (20–180)[a]	160 (50–210)
aPTT (s)	27 (20–45)	34 (25–50)	30 (20–55)
Serum lipase (U/L)	140 (60–190)	250 (140–1200)[a]	200 (135–1000)
Serum potassium (mmol/L)	4.1 (3.5–4.7)	3.4 (3.1–3.9)[a]	4.4. (4.0–5.2)
Serum sodium (mmol/L)	139 (134–145)	140 (138–150)	145 (139–155)
Creatinine clearance (mL/min/m^2)	81 (60–100)	65 (45–90)	70 (45–95)
Norepinephrine (μg/kg/min)	0	0.32 (0.0–0.45)[a]	0.08 (0.0–0.24)

aPTT, Activated partial thromboplastin time.
[a]$p < 0.05$ compared to baseline value.

not been reported so far in patients treated with mild or moderate hypothermia following head trauma or stroke. A decrease in platelet counts during the cooling period often can be seen, with recovery only after rewarming.

It is well known that hypothermia affects virtually every organ system. It has been reported in animal studies that toxicity from moderate hypothermia increases as the temperature is further decreased and as the duration of hypothermia is increased *(46,47)*. In traumatic brain injury studies by Clifton et al. *(48)* and by Marion et al. *(38)*, there were no significant increases in the number of patients with pneumonia or other infections in hypothermic or normothermic groups. On the other hand, other authors have reported an increased incidence of pneumonia after moderate, induced hypothermia *(49,50)*. Impairment of pulmonary gas exchange, caused by atelectasis, is a commonly encountered problem in patients who are ventilated for a longer time period. The reported incidence of pneumonia in these patients ranges from 10% to 40% *(51,52)*. The risk of developing pneumonia increases when coma, trauma, or impaired airway reflexes are present at admission to the critical care unit. The 40% incidence of pneumonia in our study of hypothermia in stroke patients is comparable to these reported data and similar to the findings of Metz et al., who observed pneumonia in 50% of their hypothermia-treated patients within the first week in the intensive care unit *(26)*. Also, pancreatitis with high serum amylase and lipase levels was observed following hypothermic therapy. Currently, the association between hypothermia and pancreatitis is poorly understood *(53)*. The pathological signs of pancreatitis with elevated levels of amylase and lipase are usually completely reversible after rewarming.

HYPOTHERMIA IN MODERATE MCA INFARCTS

Until now there have been very limited data on the use of hypothermia in moderate stroke. Naritomi and co-workers reported their findings of seven patients treated with hypothermia within the first 6 h after stroke onset *(54)*. Inclusion criteria for this study were embolic occlusion of the MCA proven with angiography or by Doppler ultrasound. The treatment protocol was similar to the others mentioned in the preceding. Six of the seven patients in this group were able to walk without support at the time of discharge. All of these six patients had either a small infarction or infarction without any mass effect on CT during or after hypothermic therapy.

A study by Georgiadis et al. *(31)* induced hypothermia (target temperature 33°C) in 14 patients with an acute anterior circulation infarction involving at least two thirds of the left MCA territory. Patients received norepinephrine via continuous intravenous infusion and were mechanically ventilated. Hypothermia was initiated 26 h after onset of symptoms as a means to control intracranial hypertension and not for neuroprotection. In that study, static cerebral autoregulation did not appear impaired in the unaffected hemisphere with the use of alpha-stat for pH maintenance. However, the main concern in patients with acute stroke is the perfusion of the affected hemisphere, specifically of the penumbra *(18)*.

It is obvious that further clinical trials are needed to establish the efficacy and feasibility of this method even in less severe ischemic stroke.

HYPOTHERMIA AFTER CARDIAC ARREST

Neuroprotection by rapidly applied hypothermia following global brain ischemia was recently demonstrated in patients who had been resuscitated after cardiac arrest *(55,56)*. In the study by Bernard et al. *(55)*, patients randomly assigned to hypothermic treatment were cooled within 2 h (33°C) after the return of spontaneous circulation (12-h duration). In that study, the odds ratio for a good outcome was 5.25 (95% confidence interval 1.47–18.76) and there were no significant differences in the frequency of adverse effects between temperature groups.

In the other study *(56)*, 275 patients were randomized to normothermia or hypothermia (32–34°C) over 24 h, with a median interval between restoration of circulation and hypothermic induction of 1.75 h. At 6 mo postinsult, the likelihood of a favorable outcome was significantly better in the hypothermia group (55%) compared to the normothermia group (39%, confidence interval 1.08–1.81). Mortality rates were similarly improved in the hypothermia group.

It is interesting to note that following spontaneous subarachnoid hemorrhage (SAH), body temperature falls and then rises immediately after the SAH-induced transient global cerebral ischemia without cardiac arrest *(57)*. This may be a natural cerebral protection mechanism activated by the body shortly after the insult.

FURTHER DIRECTIONS FOR HYPOTHERMIA IN STROKE

In conclusion, induced, moderate hypothermia can decrease ICP, reduce mortality, and may improve outcome in patients with severe MCA infarction with "malignant" postischemic brain edema. Important side effects are reduction of platelet count, increased rate of pneumonia, and elevation of serum amylase and lipase levels. The results of our own pilot trial suggest a beneficial effect of moderate hypothermia in the treatment of severe space-occupying MCA infarction. However, our data call for a randomized trial of hypothermia in the therapy of malignant MCA infarction. Whether early hypothermic therapy within the first 6 h after onset of symptoms can reduce infarct size has to be clarified in further clinical trials.

REFERENCES

1. Azzimondi G., Bassein L., Nonino F., et al. (1995) Fever in acute stroke worsens prognosis. A prospective study. *Stroke* **26**, 2040–2043.
2. Reith J., Jorgensen H. S., Pedersen P. M., et al. (1996) Body temperature in acute stroke: relation to stroke severity, infarct size, mortality, and outcome. *Lancet* **347**, 422–425.
3. Davalos A., Castillo J., Pumar J. M., and Noya M. (1997) Body temperature and fibrinogen are related to early neurological deterioration in acute ischemic stroke. *Cerebrovasc. Dis.* **7**, 64–69.

 4. Castillo J., Davalos A., and Noya M. (1997) Progression of ischaemic stroke and excitotoxic aminoacids. *Lancet* **349,** 79–83.
 5. Macko R. F., Ameriso S. F., Barndt R., Clough W., Weiner J. M., and Fisher M. (1996) Precipitants of brain infarction. Roles of preceding infection/inflammation and recent psychological stress. *Stroke* **27,** 1999–2004.
 6. Stone J. G., Goodman R. R., Baker K. Z., Baker C. J., and Solomon R. A. (1997) Direct intraoperative measurement of human brain temperature. *Neurosurgery* **41,** 20–24.
 7. Crowder C. M., Tempelhoff R., Theard M. A., Cheng M. A., Todorov A., and Dacey R. G., Jr. (1996) Jugular bulb temperature: comparison with brain surface and core temperatures in neurosurgical patients during mild hypothermia. *J. Neurosurg.* **85,** 98–103.
 8. Henker R. A., Brown S. D., and Marion D. W. (1998) Comparison of brain temperature with bladder and rectal temperatures in adults with severe head injury. *Neurosurgery* **42,** 1071–1075.
 9. Rumana C. S., Gopinath S. P., Uzura M., Valadka A. B., and Robertson C. S. (1998) Brain temperature exceeds systemic temperature in head-injured patients. *Crit. Care Med.* **26,** 562–567.
10. Busto R., Dietrich W. D., Globus M. Y., and Ginsberg M. D. (1989) The importance of brain temperature in cerebral ischemic injury. *Stroke* **20,** 1113–1114.
11. Schwab S., Spranger M., Aschoff A., Steiner T., and Hacke W. (1997) Brain temperature monitoring and modulation in patients with severe MCA infarction. *Neurology* **48,** 762–767.
12. Mellergard P. and Nordstrom C. H. (1991) Intracerebral temperature in neurosurgical patients. *Neurosurgery* **28,** 709–713.
13. Ko K., Ghajar J., and Hariri R. J. (1994) A method for monitoring intracranial temperature via tunneled ventricular catheter: technical note. *Neurosurgery* **34,** 927–929; discussion 929–930.
14. Nurse S. and Corbett D. (1994) Direct measurement of brain temperature during and after intraischemic hypothermia: correlation with behavioral, physiological, and histological endpoints. *J. Neurosci.* **14,** 7726–7734.
15. Haraldseth O., Gronas T., Southon T., et al. (1992) The effects of brain temperature on temporary global ischaemia in rat brain. A 31-phosphorous NMR spectroscopy study. *Acta Anaesthesiol. Scand.* **36,** 393–399.
16. Sutton L. N., Clark B. J., Norwood C. R., Woodford E. J., and Welsh F. A. (1991) Global cerebral ischemia in piglets under conditions of mild and deep hypothermia. *Stroke* **22,** 1567–1573.
17. Swain J. A., McDonald T. J., Jr., Balaban R. S., and Robbins R. C. (1991) Metabolism of the heart and brain during hypothermic cardiopulmonary bypass. *Ann. Thorac. Surg.* **51,** 105–109.
18. Ginsberg M. D. (2003) Adventures in the pathophysiology of brain ischemia: penumbra, gene expression, neuroprotection: the 2002 Thomas Willis Lecture. *Stroke* **34,** 214–223.
19. Piepgras A., Roth H., Schurer L., et al. (1998) Rapid active internal core cooling for induction of moderate hypothermia in head injury by use of an extracorporeal heat exchanger. *Neurosurgery* **42,** 311–317; discussion 317–318.
20. Jiang J. Y., Lyeth B. G., Clifton G. L., Jenkins L. W., Hamm R. J., and Hayes R. L. (1991) Relationship between body and brain temperature in traumatically brain-injured rodents. *J. Neurosurg.* **74,** 492–496.

21. Busto R., Globus M. Y., Dietrich W. D., Martinez E., Valdes I., and Ginsberg M. D. (1989) Effect of mild hypothermia on ischemia-induced release of neurotransmitters and free fatty acids in rat brain. *Stroke* **20,** 904–910.

22. Clifton G. L., Jiang J. Y., Lyeth B. G., Jenkins L. W., Hamm R. J., and Hayes R. L. (1991) Marked protection by moderate hypothermia after experimental traumatic brain injury. *J. Cereb. Blood Flow Metab.* **11,** 114–121.

23. Leonov Y., Sterz F., Safar P., et al. (1990) Mild cerebral hypothermia during and after cardiac arrest improves neurologic outcome in dogs. *J. Cereb. Blood Flow Metab.* **10,** 57–70.

24. Boris-Möller F., Smith M.-L., and Siesjo B. K. (1989) Effect of hypothermia on ischemic brain damage: a comparison between preischemic and postischemic cooling. *Neurosci. Res. Commun.* **5,** 87–94.

25. Mellergard P. (1992) Changes in human intracerebral temperature in response to different methods of brain cooling. *Neurosurgery* **31,** 671–677; discussion 677.

26. Metz C., Holzschuh M., Bein T., et al. (1996) Moderate hypothermia in patients with severe head injury: cerebral and extracerebral effects [see comments]. *J. Neurosurg.* **85,** 533–541.

27. Kurz A., Sessler D. I., Birnbauer F., Illievich U. M., and Spiss C. K. (1995) Thermoregulatory vasoconstriction impairs active core cooling. *Anesthesiology* **82,** 870–876.

28. Steinberg G. K., Ogilvy C. S., Giannotta S., et al. (2001) Multi-center trial of a venous catheter for temperature control during aneurysm surgery: preliminary review of the T. C. A. S study. *Annu. Meet. Congr. Neurol. Surg. Progr.* **51,** 255.

29. Steinberg G. K., Bell-Stephens T., Shuer L. M., et al. (2003) Comparison of endovascular cooling to surface-cooling during unrupted cerebral aneurysm repair. *Stroke,* in press.

30. De Georgia M. A., Abou-Chebl A., Krieger D. W., Andrefsky J. C., Sila C. A., and Furlan A. J. (2002) Endovascular cooling for patients with acute ischemic stroke. *Stroke* **33,** 271.

31. Georgiadis D., Schwarz S., Evans D. H., Schwab S., and Baumgartner R. W. (2002) Cerebral autoregulation under moderate hypothermia in patients with acute stroke. *Stroke* **33,** 3026–3029.

32. Hitchcock D. R., Strobel C. J. A., Haglin J. J., and Wilson J. A. (1962) Use of prolonged moderate hypothermia in postoperative care. *Arch. Surg.* **85,** 549–556.

33. Hacke W., Schwab S., Horn M., Spranger M., De Georgia M., and von Kummer R. (1996) 'Malignant' middle cerebral artery territory infarction: clinical course and prognostic signs. *Arch. Neurol.* **53,** 309–315.

34. Muizelaar J. P., Marmarou A., Ward J. D., et al. (1991) Adverse effects of prolonged hyperventilation in patients with severe head injury: a randomized clinical trial. *J. Neurosurg.* **75,** 731–739.

35. Kaufmann A. M. and Cardoso E. R. (1992) Aggravation of vasogenic cerebral edema by multiple-dose mannitol. *J. Neurosurg.* **77,** 584–589.

36. Schwab S., Spranger M., Schwarz S., and Hacke W. (1997) Barbiturate coma in severe hemispheric stroke: useful or obsolete? *Neurology* **48,** 1608–1613.

37. Schwab S., Rieke K., Aschoff A., Albert F., von Kummer R., and Hacke W. (1996) Hemicraniectomy in space-occupying hemispheric infarction: useful intervention or desperate activism? *Cerebrovasc. Dis.* **6,** 325–329.

38. Marion D. W., Penrod L. E., Kelsey S. F., et al. (1997) Treatment of traumatic brain injury with moderate hypothermia. *N. Engl. J. Med.* **336,** 540–546.

39. Ausman J. I., McCormick P. W., Stewart M., et al. (1993) Cerebral oxygen metabolism during hypothermic circulatory arrest in humans. *J. Neurosurg.* **79,** 810–815.

40. Chiara O., Giomarelli P. P., Biagioli B., Rosi R., and Gattinoni L. (1987) Hyper-metabolic response after hypothermic cardiopulmonary bypass. *Crit. Care Med.* **15,** 995–1000.
41. Aibiki M., Kawaguchi S. and Maekawa N. (2001) Reversible hypophosphatemia during moderate hypothermia therapy for brain-injured patients. *Crit. Care Med.* **29,** 1726–1730.
42. Reed R. L., 2nd, Johnson T. D., Hudson J. D., and Fischer R. P. (1992) The disparity between hypothermic coagulopathy and clotting studies. *J. Trauma* **33,** 465–470.
43. Valeri C. R., Feingold H., Cassidy G., Ragno G., Khuri S., and Altschule M. D. (1987) Hypothermia-induced reversible platelet dysfunction. *Ann. Surg.* **205,** 175–181.
44. Resnick D. K., Marion D. W., and Darby J. M. (1994) The effect of hypothermia on the incidence of delayed traumatic intracerebral hemorrhage. *Neurosurgery* **34,** 252–255; discussion 255–256.
45. Rohrer M. J. and Natale A. M. (1992) Effect of hypothermia on the coagulation cascade. *Crit. Care Med.* **20,** 1402–1405.
46. Steen P. A., Soule E. H., and Michenfelder J. D. (1979) Detrimental effect of prolonged hypothermia in cats and monkeys with and without regional cerebral ischemia. *Stroke* **10,** 522–529.
47. Michenfelder J. D. and Milde J. H. (1977) Failure of prolonged hypocapnia, hypothermia, or hypertension to favorably alter acute stroke in primates. *Stroke* **8,** 87–91.
48. Clifton G. L., Miller E. R., Choi S. C., et al. (2001) Lack of effect of induction of hypothermia after acute brain injury. *N. Engl. J. Med.* **344,** 556–563.
49. Ishikawa K., Tanaka H., Shiozaki T., et al. (2000) Characteristics of infection and leukocyte count in severely head-injured patients treated with mild hypothermia. *J. Trauma* **49,** 912–922.
50. Shiozaki T., Hayakata T., Taneda M., et al. (2001) A multicenter prospective randomized controlled trial of the efficacy of mild hypothermia for severely head injured patients with low intracranial pressure. Mild Hypothermia Study Group in Japan. *J. Neurosurg.* **94,** 50–54.
51. Chevret S., Hemmer M., Carlet J., and Langer M. (1993) Incidence and risk factors of pneumonia acquired in intensive care units. Results from a multicenter prospective study on 996 patients. European Cooperative Group on Nosocomial Pneumonia. *Intens. Care Med.* **19,** 256–264.
52. Ruiz-Santana S., Garcia Jimenez A., Esteban A., et al. (1987) ICU pneumonias: a multi-institutional study. *Crit. Care Med.* **15,** 930–932.
53. Foulis A. K. (1982) Morphological study of the relation between accidental hypothermia and acute pancreatitis. *J. Clin. Pathol.* **35,** 1244–1248.
54. Naritomi H., Shimizu T., and Oe H. (1996) Mild hypothermia therapy in acute embolic stroke: a pilot study. *J. Stroke Cerebrovasc. Dis.* **6,** 193–196.
55. Bernard S. A., Gray T. W., Buist M. D., et al. (2002) Treatment of comatose survivors of out-of-hospital cardiac arrest with induced hypothermia. *N. Engl. J. Med.* **346,** 557–563.
56. (No authors listed) (2002) The hypothermia after cardiac arrest study group: mild therapeutic hypothermia to improve the neurologic outcome after cardiac arrest. *N. Engl. J. Med.* **346,** 549–556.
57. Takagi K., Tsuchiya Y., Okinaga K., Hirata M., Nakagomi T., and Tamura A. (2003) Natural hypothermia immediately after transient global cerebral ischemia induced by spontaneous subarachnoid hemorrhage. *J. Neurosurg.* **98,** 50–56.

10 Hypothermia Therapy

Future Directions in Research and Clinical Practice

Wataru Kakuda, MD, *Takao Shimizu,* MD, *and Hiroaki Naritomi,* MD

In this chapter, we discuss the relationship between the body temperature and clinical outcome in acute stroke patients and describe our experience with the clinical application of mild hypothermia for the treatment of acute stroke. Finally, we comment on the future direction of hypothermic research and clinical practice.

CHANGES IN BODY TEMPERATURE FOLLOWING STROKE

Body temperature appears to increase rather commonly in acute stroke patients. Azzimondi et al. reported that 43% of stroke patients had a mild fever during the first 7 d after stroke *(1)*. In the study of Reith et al. *(2)*, 25% of stroke patients showed body temperature higher than 37.5°C at admission. Likewise, in the study of Hindfelt *(3)*, 48 out of 110 ischemic stroke patients had a body temperature exceeding 37.5°C during the first 7 d after stroke. These studies included patients with bacterial infections showing inflammatory reactions in laboratory tests. Therefore, fever following stroke may be attributable mainly to infectious diseases and may be unrelated to cerebral damages. However, several facts suggest that a poststroke fever may result from the cerebral injury. According to the study of Hindfelt *(3)*, fever was rarely observed in lacunar stroke, while it was commonly encountered in embolic stroke patients. We retrospectively studied changes in body temperature following acute embolic stroke of the middle cerebral artery (MCA)

From: *Hypothermia and Cerebral Ischemia: Mechanisms and Clinical Applications*
Edited by: C. M. Maier and G. K. Steinberg © Humana Press Inc., Totowa, NJ

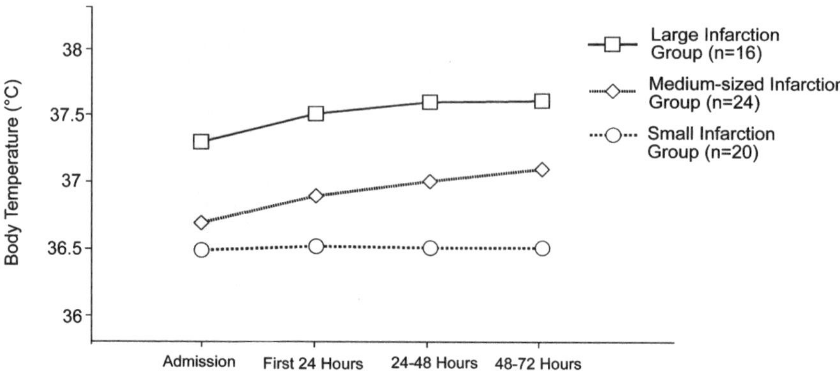

Fig. 1. Relationship between size of infarction and body temperature during the acute phase of cardiogenic embolism. Analyzed using ANOVA, the difference in body temperature among the groups was statistically significant at any period during the first 3 d after of admission.

territory in 60 patients who had no clinical or laboratory findings suggestive of infectious complications. The patients were divided into three groups according to the size of infarction on computed tomography (CT) obtained in the chronic phase: a small infarction group ($n = 20$) showing a low-density area restricted either in the basal ganglia or the cerebral cortex and subcortex, a medium-sized infarction group ($n = 24$) with a low-density area involving both the basal ganglia and cerebral cortex, and a large infarction group ($n = 16$) with a low-density area occupying the entire MCA territory. As shown in **Fig. 1**, the average body temperature during the first 3 d after stroke was $36.5 \pm 0.5°C$ in the small infarction group, $36.9 \pm 0.4°C$ in the medium-sized infarction group, and $37.5 \pm 0.6°C$ in the large infarction group, respectively. The difference in average body temperature was statistically significant ($p < 0.05$). Thus, body temperature during the first 3 d after embolic stroke increased, correlating with the size of the infarction. The fever ensued for more than 5 d in the large infarction group, while no elevation of body temperature was observed throughout the acute phase in the small infarction group. The results suggest that the involvement of a wide area of the forebrain due to stroke may lead to a fever irrespective of infectious complications.

Recently, Szczudlik et al. *(4)* studied 152 patients with supratentorial primary intracerebral hemorrhage (PICH) confirmed by CT on admission. In that study, outcome was measured by either mortality or Barthel

Index functional status 30 d after stroke. The results showed that only the severity of neurological deficit predicted greater 30-d mortality in these patients. Patients with hyperthermia on the first day of hospitalization had increased mortality and worse functional status at 30 d, but increased temperature was not an independent predictor of mortality 30 d after PICH. In a study to assess typical early onset complications following ischemic stroke, Weimar et al. *(5)* looked at a cohort of 3866 patients from 14 neurology departments with an acute stroke unit. In the first week following admission, increased intracranial pressure (ICP) and recurrent cerebral ischemia were the most frequent complications, along with fever, severe hypertension, and pneumonia. Similar concerns are also found in cardiac surgery patients in whom perioperative stroke occurred *(6)*.

These clinical results are in accordance with experimental findings on rat cerebral ischemia. In recent years, several experimental workers studied changes in body temperature following cerebral ischemia in rats under nonanesthetic conditions. Colbourne et al. *(7)* found a difference between local brain temperature and rectal temperature in the early phase of cerebral ischemia. Following cerebral ischemia, the brain temperature in the ischemic area decreased immediately, while the rectal temperature increased to approx 39°C 2–3 h thereafter. Uchino et al. *(8)* reported that the peritoneal temperature exceeded 38°C during 24 h following transient cerebral ischemia in spite of early establishment of complete recirculation. Thus, in experimental cerebral ischemia, the body core temperature increases rather commonly preceded by a decrease in cerebral temperature provided the experiments are performed under nonanesthetic conditions. To clarify the mechanisms of postischemic fever, Zhao et al. *(9)* occluded the MCA in rats using intraluminal filaments and investigated the relationship between the site of ischemic lesions and the elevation of rectal temperature. The rectal temperature increased to more than 39.0°C at 2–4 h after occlusion in spite of early establishment of recirculation. The majority of rats showing an abnormal increase in rectal temperature had ischemic damage in the ipsilateral hypothalamus. Uchino et al. *(8)* reported the same findings in rats. These authors commented that ischemic damage in the hypothalamus might be responsible for the postischemic fever in rats. It has been considered for years that the hypothalamus may be a thermoregulatory center. The obstruction of arteries supplying the hypothalamus caused by intraluminal insertion of filaments into the carotid artery likely reduces the local temperature in the hypothalamus. The local hypothermia in the thermoregulatory center may erroneously lead to the elevation of body temperature. Whether or not this view is correct, body temperature may increase following cerebral ischemia irrespective of infection.

The middle cerebral artery occlusion model (MCAO) is commonly used in experimental focal cerebral ischemia. This technique causes hypothalamic injury resulting in hyperthermia, worsening outcome and possibly masking neuroprotective effects. Thus, careful temperature monitoring is needed in those preclinical studies. Recently, Gerriets et al. *(10)* introduced a new MCAO model that involves intraarterial embolization using macrospheres. Unlike the traditional MCAO suture model, this macrosphere model does not result in hyperthermia and yet provides reproducible infarcts.

EFFECTS OF HYPERTHERMIA ON STROKE OUTCOME

The fact that profound hypothermia potentially protects the brain from ischemic insults has been known for many years. On the other hand, the effect of hyperthermia on ischemic brain was not fully recognized until the late 1980s. In 1987, Busto et al. *(11)* noticed that even a mild elevation in body temperature significantly aggravated ischemic neuronal injury in experimental animals. Dietrich et al. *(12)* found that the hyperthermia worsened ischemic blood–brain barrier (BBB) disruption, leading correlatively to the aggravation of neuronal injury. Following these reports, several clinical workers confirmed deleterious effects of hyperthermia on ischemic brain in stroke patients. Reith et al. *(2)* studied the relationships of body temperature in the acute phase of stroke with the initial stroke severity, infarct size, and clinical outcome in 1197 patients. Body temperature was significantly correlated with the initial stroke severity, infarct size, and clinical outcome. Likewise, Azzimondi et al. *(1)* and Hindfelt *(3)* found that stroke patients with fever in the acute phase had worse clinical outcomes than those without fever. Other studies have also confirmed that elevated body temperature worsens outcome and increases mortality in acute stroke patients *(13–15)*.

We studied the relationship between body temperature in the acute phase and CT findings in 60 patients with cardiogenic embolism of the MCA territory who were admitted within 24 h of stroke. Patients with an average temperature below 36.5°C during the first 3 d after admission

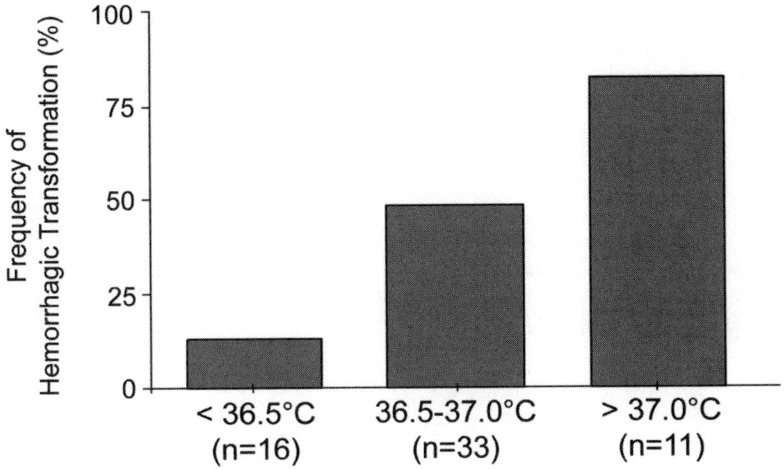

Fig. 2. Relationship between body temperature and hemorrhagic Transformation. Patients were divided into three groups according to the average value of body temperature during the first 3 d after admission. The difference in frequency among the groups was statistically significant by χ^2 tests with $p < 0.05$.

rarely had a hemorrhagic transformation on CT during the first 2 wk after admission. On the other hand, patients with an average temperature exceeding 37.0°C frequently had a hemorrhagic transformation (**Fig. 2**). Likewise, patients with an average temperature below 36.5°C rarely developed a severe cerebral edema during the first 2 wk after admission, whereas those with a fever exceeding 37.0°C commonly developed a severe cerebral edema on CT showing a shift of midline structure toward the contralateral hemisphere (**Fig. 3**). Thus, our findings are in accordance with the experimental results of Dietrich et al. *(12)* showing that hyperthermia aggravates ischemic BBB damage.

In a prospective study of 725 consecutive patients, 584 with cerebral infarcts and 141 with intracerebral hemorrhages, admitted to an acute stroke unit within 6 h of stroke onset, Boysen and Christensen measured body temperature on admission and every 2 h during the first 24 h after stroke onset *(16)*. They found that, in patients with a major stroke (defined as having a Scandinavian Stroke Scale Score ≤25), a significant rise in temperature occurred hours after stroke onset. While severe infarcts and intracerebral hemorrhages caused temperature rises, elevated body temperature on admission within 6 h of stroke onset had no prognostic influence on stroke outcome at 3 mo. It is important to

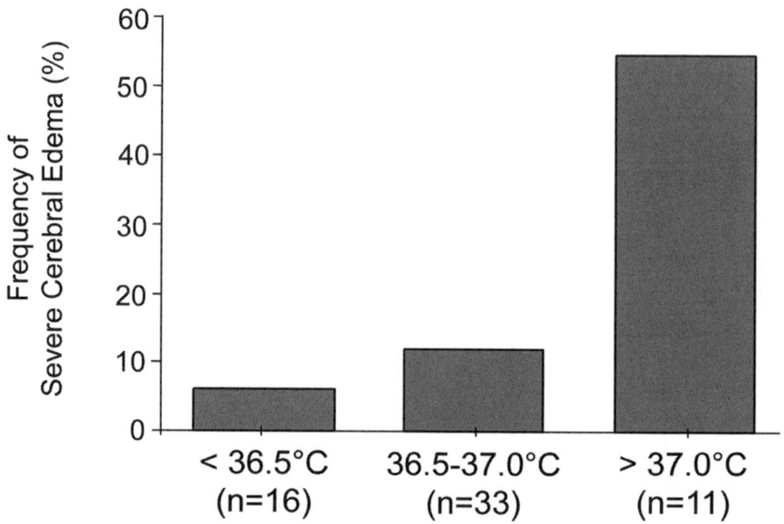

Fig. 3. Relationship between body temperature and severe cerebral edema. Patients were divided into three groups according to the average value of body temperature during the first 3 d after admission. The difference in frequency among the groups was statistically significant by χ^2 tests with $p < 0.05$.

note, however, that the initial temperature in those patients, particularly in those with severe strokes, may have been slightly below normal, as shown later by correlations of tympanic vs rectal temperature measurements *(17)*.

It is interesting to note that, in the experimental setting, hyperthermic preconditioning has been suggested as a method for inducing ischemic tolerance *(18)*.

MILD HYPOTHERMIA THERAPY IN ACUTE STROKE

Experimental Findings

A profound or moderate hypothermia below 20°C or 30°C in body temperature has been known to protect the brain from ischemic insults for many years. Profound or moderate hypothermia is, however, almost exclusively accompanied by serious cardiac suppression or other adverse effects, and hence regarded as inappropriate as a therapeutic tool except for the purpose of cerebral protection during open-heart surgery. In 1989, Busto et al. *(19)* reported that mild hypothermia in the range of 30–33°C exerted potentially protective effects on neuronal cells in experimental cerebral ischemia. Following the report, numerous researchers have confirmed the findings of Busto et al. and clarified further that mild hypothermia suppresses tissue acidosis *(20)* and lipid peroxidation *(21)* in ischemic brain, ameliorates ischemic BBB injury *(12)*, and diminishes the size of infarction produced by MCA occlusion *(22,23)*. Experimental findings are described in detail in Chapter 3.

Considerations

In spite of the accumulation of experimental data concerning beneficial effects of mild hypothermia on cerebral ischemia, hypothermia has rarely been utilized for the treatment of acute stroke. Mild hypothermia is advantageous over profound or moderate hypothermia as a tool of stroke therapy because it has fewer adverse effects on the circulatory and immunological systems. A number of investigators reported the safety and effectiveness of mild hypothermia in patients with severe head injury *(24–27)*. More recently, however, results from a large clinical trial on hypothermia and traumatic brain injury were disappointing *(28)*. That study has been criticized for potentially missing the therapeutic window for treatment with hypothermia because the target temperature was reached only after an average of approx 8.5 h after injury. Two large positive clinical trials of hypothermia for cardiac arrest have shown significant benefit with the use of this therapy *(29,30)*. Kammersgaard et al. *(31)* surface cooled 17 acute stroke patients (mean of 35.5°C) over 6 h and found that reducing temperature was not only feasible, but was also not associated with poor outcome. Smaller temperature reductions may also prove to be beneficial, although more studies are warranted in this area *(32)*. Therefore, it is reasonable to utilize mild hypothermia for the treatment of acute embolic stroke, particularly because clinical outcome of embolic stroke appears to be largely determined by the body temperature *(33)*.

Indications for Mild Hypothermia Therapy

General anesthesia is needed to perform hypothermia therapy. Without general anesthesia, the cerebral temperature cannot be lowered satisfactorily because of shivering, which usually starts at levels of 35°C. The requirement of anesthesia limits the indications for therapy. From an ethical viewpoint, general anesthesia may be permitted only in patients with consciousness disturbance. Hypothermia may be best indicated for patients with embolic occlusion of major cerebral arteries, as they usually have consciousness disturbance and their clinical outcome appears to be largely influenced by body temperature. Furthermore, the therapy may be best indicated for patients who have not yet developed ischemic changes on CT, as the value of hypothermia is to protect the brain from ischemic insults. We have been treating stroke patients with mild hypothermia since 1996 *(34)*. In our department, the therapy is indicated for patients satisfying the following criteria: (1) age <75 yr, (2) admission within 4 h after stroke, (3) consciousness disturbance and hemiparesis, (4) embolic occlusion of major cerebral artery as judged by angiography or duplex echo sonography, (5) no improvement of neurologic symptoms for more than 30 min after injection of tissue plasminogen activator (t-PA), and (6) no severe cardiac or renal dysfunction. We are, however, occasionally performing the therapy in patients who had stroke for more than 6 h prior to the therapy, provided the patient's family requests the therapy.

Hypothermic Procedure

The therapy is initiated with induction of anesthesia with diazepam and midazolam followed by intubation and artificial respiration. Prior to the anesthesia, a sufficient volume of plasma expander needs to be infused intravenously to avoid a marked drop of blood pressure, which occurs inevitably at the induction of anesthesia. The infusion of catecholamines is not appropriate for the prevention of hypotension, as catecholamines cause peripheral vasoconstriction, which disturbs body core cooling. The brain temperature is monitored with a small thermister inserted into the internal jugular bulb, and the body core temperature is monitored with a thermister placed in the bladder. According to the literature, the brain temperature is somewhat higher than the core temperature. In our experience, however, the brain temperature and bladder temperature are virtually the same. Therefore, bladder temperature monitoring alone may be satisfactory for proceeding with hypothermia therapy. The body is cooled using a commercially available hypothermic blanket in combination with an alcohol compress. In this way, the brain temperature can be lowered to 33°C within 2 h. After a target temperature is achieved, extremities should be kept warm to avoid frostbite. The brain temperature of 33°C is maintained for 3–5 d followed by rewarming and discontinuation of anesthesia. Rewarming should take more than 24 h to avoid adverse effects.

During the hypothermic period, patients are under general anesthesia, so that neurological examinations are useless for evaluating the development of cerebral infarction or cerebral edema. The electro-encephalogram (EEG) is markedly suppressed owing to the effects of hypothermia and anesthesia, and does not reflect the neurologic state adequately. Therefore, serial CT studies are needed to evaluate the development of ischemic changes, hemorrhagic changes, and cerebral edema. Duplex echo sonography and transcranial Doppler studies are quite helpful for detecting recanalization of arteries. During the hypothermic period, cardiac arrhythmias may be observed occasionally. Arrhythmias usually become prominent when the cerebral temperature is decreased below 32.5°C. Therefore, the cerebral temperature may be maintained in a range between 32.5°C and 33.4°C. Laboratory tests commonly show a progressive decrease of platelet counts during the hypothermic period. The platelet counts, however, increase rapidly after the discontinuation of hypothermia. An optimal duration for hypothermia has not yet been determined. An excessively long hypothermia period such as more than 6–7 d increases the risk of severe infection resulting from immunosuppressive effects. On the other hand, an excessively short hypothermic treatment may not protect the brain satisfactorily. Our results suggest that 3–5 d of hypothermia may be sufficient to protect the ischemic brain. Provided CT at the second or third hypothermic day shows no abnormal lesion or a small lesion, 3 d may be sufficient as a hypothermic duration. In such cases, hypothermia is considered to rescue the majority of neurons in the ischemic area from death, and no expansion of ischemic area may result. On the other hand, if CT displays a large lesion without noticeable mass effect, 5 d may be needed as a hypothermic duration. In such cases, hypothermia probably failed to rescue the majority of neurons from ischemic death, but succeeded in preserving the BBB. Discontinuation of hypothermia after a 5-d period is unlikely to be followed by the development of edema in such cases. However, if CT exhibits a large lesion in association with definitive mass effects, more than 5 d may be needed as a hypothermic duration. In such cases, the therapy probably failed to rescue neurons and failed to protect the BBB. Hypothermia may be continued until the resolution of severe edema and mass effects in such cases, although various adverse effects may accompany the continuation of hypothermia.

Hypothermic Effects on Embolic Stroke

Schwab et al. *(35)* reported the effect of mild hypothermia on acute stroke patients. They lowered the core temperature to 33°C for 2–3 d in 25 patients with large MCA territory infarction and studied the effect of mild hypothermia on clinical outcome and ICP. Hypothermia significantly decreased the ICP during the hypothermic period, although the pressure increased again after rewarming. As a consequence, 44% of patients died in spite of the therapy. Schwab et al. described this mortality to be significantly lower than in patients without mild hypothermia and commented on the usefulness of mild hypothermia for the treatment of malignant MCA territory stroke *(35)*. However, a mortality of 44% is considered too high to conclude that the therapy is effective; even though the clinical outcome of large MCA territory infarction is generally poor. Schwab et al. initiated hypothermia therapy at 14 ± 7 h after stroke, at which time the CT displayed a large ischemic change including early signs *(35)*. It is likely that the potential effect of hypothermia is largely diminished by such a delayed initiation. At 14 h after stroke, the majority of neuronal cells in the ischemic area are probably destined to die. In such circumstances, hypothermia may be unable to protect neuronal cells and may exert only suppressive effects on cerebral edema.

In our institute, we treated 14 patients with embolic occlusion of the internal carotid artery (ICA), MCA trunk, or basilar artery with mild hypothermia according to the protocol described in the preceding. All the patients were unconscious and had a hemiparesis or quadriparesis in association with ocular conjugate deviation prior to the therapy. The therapy was initiated within 6 h after stroke in 11 patients (hyperacute group) and 10–42 h in the other three patients (acute group). In the hyperacute group, the NIH Stroke Scale prior to the therapy was 22.4 ± 9.6. Nine of these patients were administered t-PA at 3.4 ± 1.6 h after stroke and showed no improvement in ischemic symptoms over 30 min. Body cooling was initiated at 4.0 ± 1.0 h after stroke and the target brain temperature of 33°C was achieved at 5.9 ± 1.4 h after stroke. The effect of hypothermia was remarkable in 9 of 11 hyperacute patients. In 8 patients, only a small or medium-sized low-density lesion developed on CT. In another patient, a large low-density lesion developed on CT; however, no mass effect was observed during the therapy and after discontinuation of therapy. The remaining two patients died during the acute phase of stroke. One of them had bilateral ICA occlusion and severe stenosis in the basilar artery, and the other one had left ICA occlusion in association with a massive hemorrhagic change on CT. The hypothermia therapy was ineffective in these two patients. Thus, the mortality in the hyperacute group was 18%. At 3 mo after stroke, all

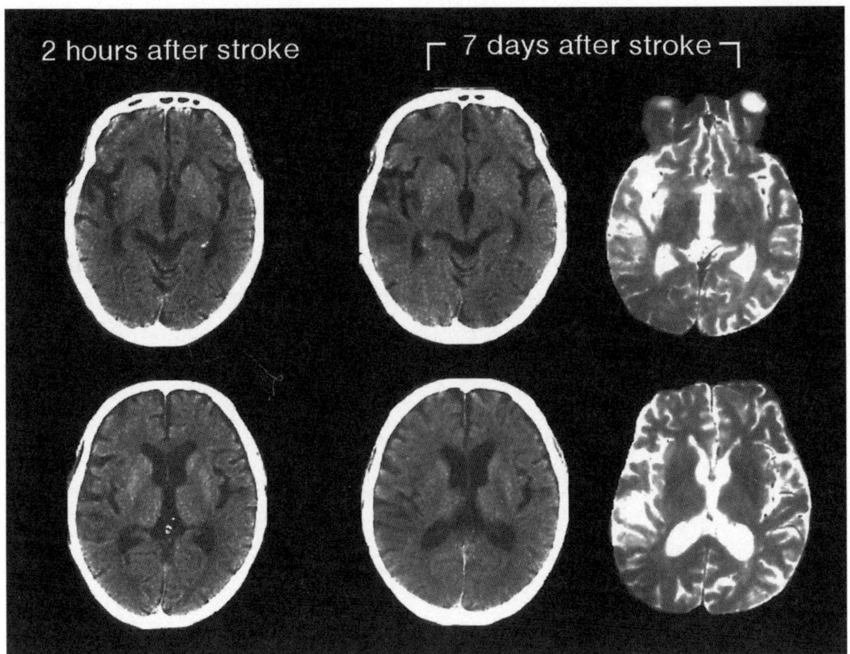

Fig. 4. CT and MRI findings in a patient undergoing hypothermia therapy in the hyperacute phase. In this patient, the hypothermia therapy was induced 4 h after embolic occlusion of the right MCA. Only a very small infarction developed in the right temporal cortex.

surviving patients except for one were able to walk with or without a cane. In these surviving patients, the average Rankin Scale at 3 mo after stroke was 2.8 ± 1.4, and the average Barthel Index at 3 mo after stroke was 75 ± 32. **Figure 4** illustrates CT and magnetic resonance imaging (MRI) findings in one case from the hyperacute group. This 68-yr-old man had the right MCA occlusion, which reopened partially 3 d after stroke. The hypothermia was induced 4 h after stroke. He developed a very small infarction in the temporal cortex. This patient had only numbness of the left fingers as a residual deficit. Thus, hypothermia therapy may be most beneficial in hyperacute stroke patients who have not yet developed ischemic changes on CT. In such patients, hypothermia may protect both neurons and the BBB, preventing the expansion of infarction and the development of cerebral edema. The fact that the majority of patients in our hyperacute group showed no contrast enhancement of ischemic lesion on CT may indicate a potential BBB protective effect of hypothermia.

In the acute group, in which the hypothermia was initiated at 10–42 h after stroke, the clinical outcome varied depending on the time of hypothermia initiation. A patient who underwent the therapy beginning at 10 h after stroke became completely independent. Another patient who underwent the therapy at 24 h after stroke had a moderate right hemiparesis, but was able to walk with a cane. The remaining patient who underwent the therapy at 42 h after stroke became disabled and died in the chronic phase. Thus, it seems that the time for initiating hypothermia critically influences the clinical outcome. This supports the view that the hypothermia therapy may be best indicated for hyperacute stroke.

PROBLEMS WITH HYPOTHERMIA THERAPY

Mild hypothermia offers a useful treatment for acute stroke. However, the therapy has several problems that may limit its wide use. The greatest problem for hypothermia therapy is a requirement for general anesthesia. Respiratory arrest, blood pressure reduction, unresponsiveness of patients, and suppression of EEG accompany general anesthesia. Accordingly, respiratory control and various drugs for maintaining optimal blood pressure levels are required. Under anesthetic conditions, a bedside evaluation of neurologic state becomes impossible, and hence frequent CT studies are needed for estimating a disease condition. Thus, patient management is complicated with hypothermia therapy and requires many well trained staff. For these reasons, the therapy may be feasibly undertaken only in a large institute with a sufficient number of experienced personnel.

Hypothermia is known to cause cardiac dysfunction, particularly arrhythmias *(36,37)*. Careful temperature control and optimal antiarrhythmic therapy can minimize this problem. However, to avoid severe circulatory dysfunction, knowledge of arrhythmias is required. Hypothermia may be associated with a suppression of the immunological system, which exposes patients to the danger of severe infections. Schwab et al. reported that 7 of 25 stroke patients undergoing hypothermia therapy suffered a septic syndrome *(17)*. In our hypothermic study, none of the 13 patients who underwent hypothermia therapy for 3–7 d developed severe infectious diseases. However, the remaining patient, who underwent 10 d of hypothermia because of massive cerebral edema, developed septic shock on the 10th day of hypothermia treatment. The immunosuppressive effect appears to be correlated with the depth and duration of hypothermia. An excessively long period of hypothermia may increase the risk of severe infections. Hypothermia may cause a coagulation abnormality or clotting abnormality *(38)*. Bleeding time was prolonged by hypothermia in baboons *(39)*, and enzymatic reactions of the coagulation cascade were inhibited by systemic hypothermia in humans *(40)*. In our study, two patients who first underwent t-PA administration developed a massive hemorrhagic transformation after the hypothermia therapy. BBB protection resulting from hypothermia may prevent the development of hemorrhagic transformation, whereas the bleeding tendency attributable to hypothermia may accelerate the development of hemorrhagic transformation. The bleeding risk may be a serious problem that should be solved in the future so as to perform the hypothermia therapy safely.

NEW CONCEPT IN HYPOTHERMIA THERAPY

The clinical use of hypothermia for the treatment of acute stroke may appear to be limited by the problems mentioned above. However, a more feasible and safer therapy might be employed. It is reasonable to consider that hypothermia ranging from 35°C to 36°C may protect the ischemic brain and exert a therapeutic effect on acute stroke, although the effect may be less beneficial than 33°C mild hypothermia. Uchino et al. *(8)* prevented the increase of body temperature following MCA occlusion in rats using an external cooling system and studied its effect on ischemic cerebral injury. This antipyretic treatment significantly decreased the frequency of postischemic seizure and ameliorated the extent of tissue damage. The results of this animal study suggest that the aggressive prevention of postischemic fever may be effective in protecting the ischemic brain. Our clinical findings in embolic stroke patients (**Figs. 2** and **3**) support the validity of this view. Core temperatures or brain temperatures of 35–36°C can be achieved by oral administration of drugs without general anesthesia. We attempted to lower the core temperature to 35–36°C in several stroke patients with mild fever by the administration of various drugs, such as indomethacin, aspirin, and chlorpromazine. In all these patients, the core temperature decreased satisfactorily below 36°C without shivering, although the blood pressure decreased in some patients and care was needed to prevent hypotension. Thus, core temperatures of 35–36°C can be achieved rather easily by administration of drugs with antipyretic actions. It is not yet clear whether such an antipyretic therapy exerts therapeutic effects on

Table 1
Comparison of Mild Hypothermia and Antipyretic Therapy

	Mild hypothermia	*Antipyretic therapy*
Target temperature	33°C	35–36°C
Protective effects	Potent	Moderate
General anesthesia	Required	Not required
Equipments	Hypothermia blanket, respirator	None
Patient management	Complicated	Easy
Indicative stroke subtype	Mainly embolic stroke	Any subtype
Indicative patients	Unconscious patients	Any patients
Neurological evaluation	Impossible	Possible
Adverse effects	Possible	Small

stroke. However, antipyretic therapy is considered worth trying, as it has advantages over mild hypothermia therapy (*see* **Table 1**). Any hospitals or physicians can utilize antipyretic therapy, as it requires no special equipment. The effectiveness of such antipyretic therapy should be evaluated in the future. Recently, a study by Knoll et al. *(32)* showed that continuous body core temperature reduction of 1–2°C may safely be attained and critically high temperature values can be avoided by a cooling mattress in nonventilated stroke unit patients. However, the neuroprotective potential of this method has yet to be assessed in a controlled clinical trial.

CURRENT INVESTIGATIONS

There is a considerable amount of research underway in the preclinical arena focusing on combining hypothermia therapy with other agents, particularly antiinflammatory drugs and free radical scavengers (for further details *see* Chapter 6). The possibility of developing animal lines with altered body core temperatures is also under investigation and may aid in the study of physiological responses to forced vs regulated hypothermia treatment *(41,42)*. As always, the optimization of any therapy depends on our understanding of the mechanisms involved in the injury or disease process.

In the clinical field, technological advances such as the development of transvenous catheters for rapid patient cooling are making implementation of hypothermia therapy more feasible and safer. More definitive trials on the use of therapeutic hypothermia are underway.

REFERENCES

1. Azzimondi G., Bassein L., Nonino F., et al. (1995) Fever in acute stroke worsens prognosis. *Stroke* **26,** 2040–2043.
2. Reith J., Jorgensen H. S., Pedersen P. M., et al. (1996) Body temperature in acute stroke: relation to stroke severity, infarct size, mortality, and outcome. *Lancet* **347,** 422–425.
3. Hindfelt B. (1976) The prognostic significance of subfebrility and fever in ischaemic cerebral infarction. *Acta Neurol. Scand.* **53,** 72–79.
4. Szczudlik A., Turaj W., Slowik A., and Strojny J. (2002) Hyperthermia is not an independent predictor of greater mortality in patients with primary intracerebral hemorrhage. *Med. Sci. Monit.* **8,** CR702–7.
5. Weimar C., Roth M. P., Zillessen G., et al. (2002) Complications following acute ischemic stroke. *Eur. Neurol.* **48,** 133–140.
6. Hindman B. J. (2002) Emboli, inflammation, and CNS impairment: an overview. *Heart Surg. Forum* **5,** 249–253.
7. Colbourne F., Nurse S. M., and Corbett D. (1993) Temperature changes associated with forebrain ischemia in the gerbil. *Brain Res.* **602,** 264–267.
8. Uchino H., Lundgren J., Smith M. L., and Siesjo B. K. (1994) Preischemic hyperglycemia leads to delayed postischemic hyperthermia. *Stroke* **25,** 1825–1829.
9. Zhao Q., Memezawa H., Smith M. L., and Siesjo B. K. (1994) Hyperthermia complicates middle cerebral artery occlusion induced by an intraluminal filament. *Brain Res.* **649,** 253–259.
10. Gerriets T., Li F., Silva M. D., Meng X., Brevard M., Sotak C. H., and Fisher M. (2003) The macrosphere model. Evaluation of a new stroke model for permanent middle cerebral artery occlusion in rats. *J. Neurosci. Methods* **122,** 201–211.
11. Busto R., Dietrich W. D., Globus M. Y., Valdes I., Scheinberg P., and Ginsberg M. D. (1987) Small differences in intraischemic brain temperature critically determine the extent of ischemic neuronal injury. *J. Cereb. Blood Flow Metab.* **7,** 729–738.
12. Dietrich W. D., Busto R., Halley M., and Valdes I. (1990) The importance of brain temperature in alterations of the blood-brain barrier following cerebral ischemia. *J. Neuropathol. Exp. Neurol.* **49,** 486–497.
13. Castillo J., Davalos A., Marrugat J., and Noya M. (1998) Timing for fever-related brain damage in acute ischemic stroke. *Stroke* **29,** 2455–2460.
14. Hajat C., Hajat S., and Sharma P. (2000) Effects of poststroke pyrexia on stroke outcome: a meta-analysis of studies in patients. *Stroke* **31,** 410–414.
15. Wang Y., Lim L. L., Levi C., Heller R. F., and Fisher J. (2000) Influence of admission body temperature on stroke mortality. *Stroke* **31,** 404–409.
16. Boysen G. and Christensen H. (2001) Stroke severity determines body temperature in acute stroke. *Stroke* **32,** 413–417.
17. Christensen H. and Boysen G. (2002) Acceptable agreement between tympanic and rectal temperature in acute stroke patients. *Int. J. Clin. Pract.* **56,** 82–84.
18. Ota A., Ikeda T., Xia X. Y., Xia Y. X., and Ikenoue T. (2000) Hypoxic–ischemic tolerance induced by hyperthermic pretreatment in newborn rats. *J. Soc. Gynecol. Invest.* **7,** 102–105.
19. Busto R., Dietrich W. D., Globus M. Y., and Ginsberg M. D. (1989) Postischemic moderate hypothermia inhibits CA1 hippocampal ischemic neuronal injury. *Neurosci. Lett.* **101,** 299–304.

20. Chopp M., Welch K. M., Tidwell C. D., Knight R., and Helpern J. A. (1988) Effect of mild hyperthermia on recovery of metabolic function after global cerebral ischemia in cats. *Stroke* **19**, 1521–1525.
21. Lei B., Tan X., Cai H., Xu Q., and Guo Q. (1994) Effect of moderate hypothermia on lipid peroxidation in canine brain tissue after cardiac arrest and resuscitation. *Stroke* **25**, 147–152.
22. Morikawa E., Ginsberg M. D., Dietrich W. D., et al. (1992) The significance of brain temperature in focal cerebral ischemia: histopathological consequences of middle cerebral artery occlusion in the rat. *J. Cereb. Blood Flow Metab.* **12**, 380–389.
23. Ridenour T. R., Warner D. S., Todd M. M., and McAllister A. C. (1992) Mild hypothermia reduces infarct size resulting from temporary but not permanent focal ischemia in rats. *Stroke* **23**, 733–738.
24. Marion D. W., Penrod L. E., Kelsey S. F., et al. (1997) Treatment of traumatic brain injury with moderate hypothermia. *N. Engl. J. Med.* **336**, 540–546.
25. Clifton G. L., Allen S., Barrodale P., et al. (1993) A phase II study of moderate hypothermia in severe brain injury. *J. Neurotrauma* **10**, 263–271; discussion 273.
26. Shiozaki T., Sugimoto H., Taneda M., et al. (1993) Effect of mild hypothermia on uncontrollable intracranial hypertension after severe head injury. *J. Neurosurg.* **79**, 363–368.
27. Metz C., Holzschuh M., Bein T., et al. (1996) Moderate hypothermia in patients with severe head injury: cerebral and extracerebral effects [see comments]. *J. Neurosurg.* **85**, 533–541.
28. Clifton G. L., Miller E. R., Choi S. C., et al. (2001) Lack of effect of induction of hypothermia after acute brain injury. *N. Engl. J. Med.* **344**, 556–563.
29. Bernard S. A., Gray T. W., Buist M. D., et al. (2002) Treatment of comatose survivors of out-of-hospital cardiac arrest with induced hypothermia. *N. Engl. J. Med.* **346**, 557–563.
30. (No authors listed) (2002) The hypothermia after cardiac arrest study group: mild therapeutic hypothermia to improve the neurologic outcome after cardiac arrest. *N. Engl. J. Med.* **346**, 549–556.
31. Kammersgaard L. P., Rasmussen B. H., Jorgensen H. S., Reith J., Weber U., and Olsen T. S. (2000) Feasibility and safety of inducing modest hypothermia in awake patients with acute stroke through surface cooling: a case-control study: the Copenhagen Stroke Study. *Stroke* **31**, 2251–2256.
32. Knoll T., Wimmer M. L., Gumpinger F., and Haberl R. L. (2002) The low normothermia concept—maintaining a core body temperature between 36 and 37 degrees C in acute stroke unit patients. *J. Neurosurg. Anesthesiol.* **14**, 304–308.
33. Thornhill J. and Corbett D. (2001) Therapeutic implications of hypothermic and hyperthermic temperature conditions in stroke patients. *Can. J. Physiol. Pharmacol.* **79**, 254–261.
34. Naritomi H., Shimizu T., and Oe H. (1996) Mild hypothermia therapy in acute embolic stroke: a pilot study. *J. Stroke Cerebrovasc. Dis.* **6**, 193–196.
35. Schwab S., Schwarz S., Aschoff A., Keller E., and Hacke W. (1998) Moderate hypothermia and brain temperature in patients with severe middle cerebral artery infarction. *Acta Neurochir. Suppl.* **71**, 131–134.
36. Laptook A. R. and Corbett R. J. (2002) The effects of temperature on hypoxic-ischemic brain injury. *Clin. Perinatol.* **29**, 623–649, vi.
37. Nussmeier N. A. (2002) A review of risk factors for adverse neurologic outcome after cardiac surgery. *J. Extracorpor. Technol.* **34**, 4–10.

38. Reed R. L., 2nd, Johnson T. D., Hudson J. D., and Fischer R. P. (1992) The disparity between hypothermic coagulopathy and clotting studies. *J. Trauma* **33,** 465–470.
39. Valeri C. R., Feingold H., Cassidy G., Ragno G., Khuri S., and Altschule M. D. (1987) Hypothermia-induced reversible platelet dysfunction. *Ann. Surg.* **205,** 175–181.
40. Rohrer M. J. and Natale A. M. (1992) Effect of hypothermia on the coagulation cascade. *Crit. Care Med.* **20,** 1402–1405.
41. Gordon C. J. and Rezvani A. H. (2001) Genetic selection of rats with high and low body temperatures. *J. Therm. Biol.* **26,** 223–229.
42. Gordon C. J. (2001) The therapeutic potential of regulated hypothermia. *Emerg. Med. J.* **18,** 81–89.

Index

A

Acetylcholine, 133
Active controls, 101
Active core cooling, 5
Acute cerebral ischemia
   pharmaceuticals
      with hypothermia, 93–101
Acute intracranial hemorrhage
   mild hypothermia, 107
Acute ischemic stroke
   clinical trial design, 100t
   endovascular cooling, 110
   mild hypothermia, 8–11
   preclinical experimental criteria,
      99t
Acute severe middle cerebral artery
      (MCA) infarction
   mild hypothermia, 107
Acute stroke
   mild hypothermia, 166–172
Alpha-amino-3-hydroxy-5-methyl-
      4-isoxazolepropionic acid
      (AMPA) antagonist, 80–81
AMPA, 80–81
Amylase, 156
Amyloid precursor protein (APP), 66
Aneurysms, 104
Animal models
   hypothermia
      experimental studies, 3–5
   variability, 3
Anoxic depolarization, 69
Antiapoptotic proteins, 57
Antiinflammatory agents, 95
Antipyretic treatment, 173–174

   vs mild hypothermia, 174t
Apoptosis, 40, 72
APP, 66
APTT
   moderate hypothermia, 155t
Arrhythmias, 104, 120, 135, 172
Artificial ventilation, 150
Aspartate, 28, 40, 133
Atelectasis, 155t
Atracurium, 151
Atrial fibrillation, 108

B

Baboons
   hypothermia complications, 154
   traumatic brain injury (TBI), 132
Balance beam, 67, 129
Barbiturates, 150
Barthel Index functional status
   primary intracerebral hemorrhage
      (PICH), 162–163
Bax, 57
Bcl-2, 57, 105
BDNF, 30
Beam-balance tasks, 67, 129
Beam-walking tasks, 67
Behavioral improvement
   posttraumatic hypothermia, 67–68
Behavioral outcome, 4
Bias
   avoidance, 100
Bladder irrigation
   warm saline, 114
Bleeding, 104
Bleeding disorders, 109
Blood-brain barrier, 54, 71, 131, 164

breakdown, 29
permeability of, 134–135
Blood clot embolization, 41
Blood pressure, 52–53
   reduction, 172
Body surface cooling, 148
Body temperature
   vs brain temperature, 146–148
      head trauma, 147
   cerebral edema, 166, 166f
   hemorrhagic transformation, 165, 165f
   infarction, 162f
   stroke, 161–164, 162
      clinical evidence, 145–146
Brain
   cooling techniques, 5–6
   temperature
      global ischemia, 19
Brain-derived neurotrophic factor (BDNF), 30
Brain injury
   hypothermia
      experimental studies, 3–5
      resurgence, 1–11
Brain temperature
   body core temperature, 146–148
   vs body core temperature
      head trauma, 147
   measurement, 146
   middle cerebral artery (MCA) infarction, 146–147
   protocol, 151
   stroke, 146–148
Brain tumors
   vascular, 104
Brief hypothermia, 80
Buspirone, 110

C

Calcium, 95, 105, 133
Calcium/calmodulin-dependent protein kinase II (CaM kinase II), 29
Calmodulin, 26
Canine epidural balloon-compression model, 129
Canine global cerebral ischemia models
   delayed postischemic hypothermia, 85
Canines
   cardiac arrest, 21
   focal cerebral ischemia
      delayed hypothermia, 86
Cardiac arrest, 9–10
   hypothermia, 156–157
      mild hypothermia, 105
      moderate hypothermia, 21
Cardiac dysfunction, 172
Cardiac rhythm, 95
Cardiopulmonary bypass
   deep hypothermia, 104
   moderate hypothermia, 21
Carotid arteries
   catheterization, 6
   occlusion
      gerbil, 81
Cats
   focal cerebral ischemic studies on, 47t
      delayed hypothermia, 86
CBF, 26–27, 52–57
   hypothermia, 123t, 124
Cerebral artery (MCA) infarction
   moderate middle hypothermia, 156
Cerebral blood flow (CBF), 26–27, 52–57
   hypothermia, 123t, 124
Cerebral edema, 54
Cerebral ischemia
   acute

pharmaceuticals with
    hypothermia, 93–101
focal models, *see* Focal cerebral
    ischemia
global models, *see* Global
    cerebral ischemia
Cerebral metabolic rate (CMR),
    52–57
Cerebral metabolic rate of oxygen
    (CMRO2)
    hypothermia, 123t, 124
Cerebral metabolism, 132–135
    hypothermia, 123t
Cerebral perfusion pressure (CPP), 6
    hypothermia, 123t
CGS-19755, 97
Children, 109–110
Clinical hypothermia, 148
    stroke, 149
Clinical trials, 106
    vs experimental studies, 4–5
Clotting abnormality, 173
CMR, 52–57
CMRO2
    hypothermia, 123t, 124
Coagulation defects, 109, 135
Cognitive deficits, 67
Cold gastric lavage, 148
Contemporary clinical studies,
    120–129
Cooled air fans, 148
Cooling blankets, 110, 151
Cooling methods, 110–112
Copenhagen group, 145
CPP, 6
    hypothermia, 123t
Craniotomy, 105
Creatinine
    moderate hypothermia, 155t
Cryoglobulinopathy, 109
Cytochrome c, 105

Cytokines, 56, 71–72
Cytotoxic edema, 54

D

Dantrolene, 105
Decompressive surgery, 150
Deep hypothermia
    cardiopulmonary bypass
      (CPB), 104
    operative setting, 103
Delayed hypothermia
    focal cerebral ischemia, 85–86
Delayed postischemic hypothermia
    canine global cerebral ischemia
      models, 85
Dextromethorphan, 97
DHBA, 29–30
Diazepam, 168
DIC, 105
Dihydroxybenzoic acid (DHBA),
    29–30
2,3-dihydroxy-6-nitro-
    7sulfamoylbenzo(F)quinoxaline
    (NBQX), 81
Disseminated intravascular
    coagulopathy (DIC), 105
Dizocilpine, 23
Dogs
    cardiac arrest, 21
    epidural balloon-compression
      model, 129
    focal cerebral ischemia
      delayed hypothermia, 86
    global cerebral ischemia models
      delayed postischemic
        hypothermia, 85
Dopamine, 105

E

EAA, 40, 53, 133–134, *see also*
    individual acids

Edema, 71
EEG
    suppression, 172
Electroencephalography (EEG)
    suppression, 172
Electrolyte balance, 95
Embolic stroke
    hypothermia, 169–172
Endovascular cooling
    acute ischemic stroke, 110
Endovascular heat exchanger, 110
Endpoints, 4–5
Epidural balloon-compression model
    canine, 129
Excitatory amino acids (EAA), 40,
        53, 133–134, *see also* indi-
        vidual acids
Excitotoxic index, 25, 28
Excitotoxicity, 70
Experimental focal cerebral is-
        chemia, 41–42
    mild hypothermia, 39–57
Experimental studies
    vs clinical trials, 4–5
Extracorporeal heat exchanger, 148
Extracorporeal bypass, 2

F

Fans, 110
Fay, Temple, 1, 103–104
Feline focal cerebral ischemic
        studies, 47t
    delayed hypothermia, 86
Fentanyl, 151
Fever, 8–9, 163
Focal cerebral ischemia, 3
    delayed hypothermia, 85–86
    feline studies, 47t
        delayed hypothermia, 86
    studies on, 42t–48t
    time window, 49–50
Focal cerebral thrombosis
    photochemically induced, 41

Focal embolic ischemia model, 98
Forebrain ischemia models, 3
Free radicals, 54–56

G

Gamma-aminobutyric acid, 25
GCS, 6
    differences, 126t
Gene expression, 30, 57, 71–72
General anesthesia, 110, 167, 172
Genetic models, 56–57
Gerbils
    carotid artery occlusion, 81
    ischemic functional impairments,
        82
    T-maze performance, 84f
Glasgow Coma Scale (GCS), 6
    differences, 126t
Glasgow Outcome Score (GOS),
        106, 122
Global cerebral ischemia, 3, 17–31
    brain temperature, 19
    canine models
        delayed postischemic
            hypothermia, 85
    delayed hypothermia
        rodents, 80–84
    mild/moderate hypothermia,
        18–21
    postischemic hypothermia, 21–24
Global transient forebrain ischemia,
        96–97
Glutamate, 25, 28, 40, 53, 105, 133
    receptor antagonist, 94
Glycerol, 150
Glycine, 25, 28
GOS, 106, 122

H

Head injuries
    body core vs brain temperature,
        147
    hypothermia, 113–114

mild hypothermia, 2, 105
Heart rate
   hypothermia, 123t
Hippocampus
   necrosis, 20f–21f
Hypertension, 163
Hyperthermia
   deleterious effect, 24–26
   stroke outcome, 164–166
Hypothermia, 145–157
   abandoned, 2, 104
   brain injury
      experimental studies, 3–5
      resurgence, 1–11
   brain scans, 171, 171f
   cardiac arrest, 156–157
   cerebral blood flow (CBF),
      123t, 124
   cerebral metabolic rate of oxygen
      (CMRO2), 123t, 124
   cerebral metabolism, 123t
   cerebral perfusion pressure
      (CPP), 123t
   combination
      acute ischemic stroke, 95t
   complications, 1–2, 104,
      154–156
   current investigations, 174
   defined, 149
   differences following, 127t
   embolic stroke, 169–172
   head injuries, 113–114
   heart rate, 123t
   history, 119–120
   malignant middle cerebral artery
      (MCA) infarcts, 150–153
   mechanisms, 131–132
   moderate middle cerebral artery
      (MCA) infarct, 156
   neuroprotection mechanisms,
      26–30, 52–57, 68–69
   new concept, 173–174
   with pharmaceuticals

   acute cerebral ischemia, 93–101
   problems, 172–173
   procedure, 168–169
   results, 151–154
   stroke, 113–114
      future, 157
   therapy, 161–174
   time window, 50f, 51f, 52
   traumatic brain injury (TBI),
      65–74
   trials
      characteristics and outcomes,
         121t

I

ICAM, 146
Ice packs, 110
ICP, 6, 120, 124–125, 153f
IGF, 97
IL-1
   RNA, 72
IL-6, 134
IL-1beta, 134
Imaging studies, 4
Immediate postischemic
   hypothermia, 80
Immune system, 40
Induced hypothermia
   history, 1–2
Infection, 135, 173
Inflammation, 54–56, 72–73
Innercool Therapies Celsius Control
   System, 110, 111f
Inspired gases, 114
Insulin-like growth factor (IGF), 97
Intensive care
   mild hypothermia, 113–114
Intercellular cell adhesion molecule
   (ICAM), 146
Interleukin-1 (IL-1)
   RNA, 72
Interleukin-6 (IL-6), 134
Interleukin-1beta (IL-1beta), 134

Intracellular energy stores, 134–135
Intracellular messengers, 28–29
Intracranial hypertension
surgery, 150
Intracranial pressure (ICP), 6, 120, 124–125, 153f
Intraischemic brain temperature
vs rectal temperature, 41
Intraischemic hypothermia, 22, 28
Intraoperative cooling, 112–113
Intraoperative management
mild hypothermia, 103–114
Intraparenchymatous temperature
monitoring, 147f
Intravenous cooling, 6
Intravenous fluids, 110
Ion channel blockers, 95
Ion homeostasis, 69–70, 133
Ischemic cascade, 40
Ischemic core, 39
necrotic cell death, 40
Ischemic functional impairments
gerbil, 82
Ischemic infarction
mild hypothermia, 107
Ischemic neuronal death, 104–105
Ischemic penumbra, 39, 40
Isoflurane, 98

K

Knockout (KO) mice, 56–57
KO mice, 56–57

L

LCBF, 27
LCMRglu, 27
Lipase, 156
moderate hypothermia, 155t
Local cerebral blood flow (LCBF), 27
Local cerebral glucose utilization
(LCMRglu), 27

M

Magnesium, 97
Malignant hyperthermia, 105
Malignant middle cerebral artery
(MCA) infarction, 149–150
hypothermia, 150–153
therapy, 150
Mannitol, 150
MCA. See Middle cerebral artery
(MCA)
Mechanical ventilation, 156
Memory impairment, 67
Meperidine, 110
Metabolism, 26–27, 95
Metastatic disease, 103–104
Microtubule-associated protein 2
(MAP2), 26, 72
Midazolam, 168
Middle cerebral artery (MCA), 9, 41
blockage, 3
Middle cerebral artery (MCA)
infarction
acute severe
mild hypothermia, 107
brain temperature, 146–147
malignant, 149–150
hypothermia, 150–153
therapy, 150
Middle cerebral artery occlusion
(MCAO), 53, 85, 164
Mild hypothermia, 2
acute intracranial hemorrhage, 107
acute ischemic stroke, 8–11
acute severe middle cerebral artery
(MCA) infarction, 107
acute stroke, 166–172
vs antipyretic treatment, 174t
cardiac arrest, 105
complications, 108–109
experimental focal cerebral
ischemia, 39–57

head injury, 2, 105
intraoperative and intensive care
    management, 103–114
ischemic infarction, 107
neuroprotective effects, 3–5
neuroprotective mechanism,
    39–40
patient selection, 109–110
with pharmacological agents, 10
severe head injury, 106–107
stroke, 2, 105
    protocol, 151t
    studies
        goals, 4
        results interpretation, 3
    surgical patients, 105
    traumatic brain injury (TBI), 6–8
Mild/moderate hypothermia
    global cerebral ischemia, 18–21
Mitochondrial dysfunction, 70–71
MK-801, 96
Moderate hypothermia
    cardiac arrest, 21
    cardiopulmonary bypass, 21
    complications resulting from,
        134–135, 135–136
    experimental evidence supporting,
        129–131
    side effects on organ systems,
        155t
    temporary arterial occlusion, 104
    traumatic brain injury (TBI),
        119–137, 130t
Moderate middle cerebral artery
    (MCA) infarction
    hypothermia, 156
Modified Levine hypoxic-ischemic
    model, 97
Monkeys
    focal cerebral ischemia
        delayed hypothermia, 86
Mortality

primary intracerebral hemorrhage
    (PICH), 162–163
Myeloperoxidase, 55, 73

N

Necrotic cell death
    ischemic core, 40
Nerve growth factor (NGF), 30
Neurofilaments, 72
Neuromuscular blocking agents,
    108, 113–114
Neuronal damage, 129
    variability, 41
Neuronal NOS (nNOS), 56
Neurotransmitters
    release, 27–28
Neurotrophin-3 (NT3), 30
New Zealand White rabbits
    focal cerebral ischemic studies
        on, 42t, 46t
NGF, 30
Nitric oxide (NO), 56, 72
NMDA antagonist, 23, 96–97
N-methyl-D-aspartate (NMDA)
    antagonist, 23, 96–97
NNOS, 56
NO, 56, 72
Norepinephrine, 156
    moderate hypothermia, 155t
NT3, 30
N-tert-butyl-alpha-phenylnitrone
    (PBN), 97
    with postischemic hypothermia, 23
Nutrition, 109

O

Operative setting
    deep hypothermia, 103
Osmotherapy, 150
Outcome measures, 4
Oxygen
    consumption, 132–135

P

Pain control, 104
Pancreatitis, 156
Pancuronium, 113
Paradoxical cooling, 112–113
Parasagittal fluid percussion (F-P)
        brain injury, 65–67
Partial thromboplastin time
        (PTT), 136
Passive rewarming, 114
PBN, 97
    with postischemic hypothermia, 23
Pethidine, 108
Pharmaceuticals
    with hypothermia
        acute cerebral ischemia, 93–101
    with mild hypothermia, 10
Photochemically induced focal
        cerebral thrombosis, 41
PKC, 28–29
Plasma expander, 168
Platelet count
    moderate hypothermia, 155t
PMN, 134
Pneumonia, 155t, 163
Polymorphonuclear leukocytes
        (PMN), 134
Postinjury moderate hypothermia, 129
Postischemic hypothermia, 30, 66
    global cerebral ischemia, 21–24
    long-term neuroprotection
        rodents, 79–87
    with *n*-tert-butyl-alpha-
        phenylnitrone (PBN), 23
    permanent neuroprotection, 22
Postischemic oxygen radical
        production, 25–26
Posttraumatic hyperthermia, 68
Posttraumatic hypothermia
    behavioral improvement, 67–68
    histopathological outcome, 65–67

Posttraumatic inflammatory process,
        134
Potassium
    moderate hypothermia, 155t
Premature ventricular contractions
        (PVC), 105
Proapoptotic proteins, 57
Propofol, 98, 133, 151
Protein kinase C (PKC), 28–29
Proteins
    synthesis, 30
PTT, 136
PVC, 105

R

Rabbits
    brain ischemia, 18
    global ischemia, 28
Rats, *see also* individual types
    embolic stroke model, 98
    focal cerebral ischemia
        delayed hypothermia, 85–86
    hyperthermia, 24–25
    myeloperoxidase (MPO), 73
    postischemic hypothermia, 27
        permanent neuroprotection, 22
    subdural hematoma model, 132
    two-vessel occlusion model, 80
RCBF, 49
Reactive oxygen species, 29–30,
        54–56, 105
Rebound intracranial hypertension,
        153
Recombinant tissue plasminogen
        activator (rt-PA), 95t
Rectal temperature
    vs intraischemic brain
        temperature, 41
Regional cerebral blood flow
        (rCBF), 49
Respiratory arrest, 172
Rewarming, 68, 114, 153

Rodents, *see also* Rats
  global cerebral ischemia
    delayed hypothermia, 80–84
  models, 129
  postischemic hypothermia
    long-term neuroprotection,
      79–87
  traumatic brain injury (TBI), 132
Room temperature, 110
Rt-PA, 95t

S

SAH, 9, 157
Saline solution, 6
SD, 69
SD rats
  focal cerebral ischemic studies
    on, 43t, 44t, 45t, 46t,
    47t, 48t
Selective brain cooling, 5
Sepsis, 135
Septic shock, 172
Septic syndrome, 172
Septum pellucidum, 154f
Severe head injury
  mild hypothermia, 106–107
Severe hypothermia, 109
Sheep
  focal cerebral ischemia
    delayed hypothermia, 85–86
Shivering, 167
  prevention, 5
  suppression, 110
SH rats
  focal cerebral ischemic studies
    on, 42t, 45t
Skin
  integrity, 109
SOD, 55
Sodium
  moderate hypothermia, 155t
SOD2-KO mice, 57

Somatosensory evoked potential
  (SSEP), 113
Spectrin, 72
Spiegelberg intraparenchymatous
  ICP probe, 151
Spreading depression (SD), 69
SSEP, 113
Stanford intraoperative mild
  hypothermia cases, 106t
Stroke
  body core temperature, 161–164
  brain temperature, 146–148
  clinical hypothermia, 149
  hypothermia, 113–114
    future, 157
  mild hypothermia, 2, 105
    protocol, 151t
  outcome, 39
    hyperthermia, 164–166
  temperature control, 148
  time window, 49
Subarachnoid hemorrhage (SAH),
  9, 157
Superoxide dismutase (SOD), 55
Surface cooling, 2
Surgical patients
  mild hypothermia, 105
Systemic surface cooling, 5

T

TAI, 66–67
TBI. See Traumatic brain injury
  (TBI)
Temperature control
  stroke, 148
Temporary arterial occlusion
  moderate hypothermia, 104
Thermoregulation, 1
Thermoregulatory vasoconstriction,
  148
Thrombolysis, 10, 98
TIA, 82

Time window
  hypothermia, 52
  stroke, 49
Tirilizad, 97
Tissue plasminogen activator (t-PA),
    10, 170
TNF, 134
T-PA, 10, 170
Transferase dUTP nick-end labeling
    (TUNEL), 72
Transient forebrain ischemia
  global model, 96–97
Transient ischemia models, 96–97
Transient ischemic attacks (TIA), 82
Transvenous catheter devices, 148
Trauma-induced axonal injury
    (TAI), 66–67
Traumatic brain injury (TBI)
  hypothermic protection, 65–74
  mild hypothermia, 6–8
  moderate hypothermia, 119–137,
    130t
TrkB, 30
Tumor necrosis factor (TNF), 134

TUNEL, 72

U

Ubiquitin, 105
University of Pittsburgh Study, 126t,
    127t

V

Vascular cell adhesion molecule
    (VCAM), 146
Vasogenic edema, 54
VCAM, 146
Ventricular fibrillation, 9–10, 120

W

Warm air blanket, 114
Warming blanket, 110
Warm saline
  bladder irrigation, 114
Water blankets, 148
Wistar rats
  brain ischemia, 19
  focal cerebral ischemic studies on,
    42t, 43t, 44t, 45t, 46t, 47t